the path of **yoga**

OSHO

Extemporaneous talks given by Osho
in Mumbai, India

the path of **yoga**

Discovering the Essence and Origin of Yoga

THE YOGA SUTRAS OF PATANJALI

OSHO

Previously published as *Yoga: The Alpha and the Omega,* Vol. 1

This book is from a series of original talks by Osho, *Yoga: The Science of the Soul,*
Vol.1, given to a live audience. All of Osho's talks have been published in full as
books, and are also available as original audio recordings. Audio recordings and the
complete text archive can be found via the online OSHO Library at
www.osho.com/library

Original sutras from *The Yoga Sutras of Patanjali* translated from Sanskrit by Yoga
Chinmaya, Copyright © 1973 OSHO International Foundation.

OSHO MEDIA INTERNATIONAL
New York • Zurich • Mumbai
an imprint of
OSHO INTERNATIONAL
www.osho.com/oshointernational

Distributed by Publishers Group Worldwide
www.pgw.com

Library of Congress Catalog-In-Publication Data is available

ISBN-13: 978-0-918963-09-3
This title is also available in eBook format ISBN: 978-0-88050-291-7

Printed in USA

contents

Preface   vi

1   Introduction to the Path of Yoga   1

2   Desireless, You Are Enlightened   23

3   Five Modifications of Mind   45

4   Madness or Meditation   71

5   Why Can't You Dance?   89

6   The Purity of Yoga   115

7   An Ecstasy Is Born   137

8   Stop, and It Is Here!   161

9   This Very Life, the Ultimate Joy   183

10   The End Is in the Beginning   205

About Osho   228

OSHO International Meditation Resort   229

For More Information   231

preface

Mind is not a thing, but an event. A thing has substance in it; an event is just a process. A thing is like a rock; an event is like a wave: it exists, but is not substantial. It is just the event between the wind and the ocean ̄ a process, a phenomenon.

This is the first thing to be understood: that mind is a process, like a wave or like a river, but it has no substance in it. If it has substance, then it cannot be dissolved. If it has no substance, it can disappear without leaving a single trace behind. When a wave disappears into the ocean what is left behind? – nothing, not even a trace. So those who have known say mind is like a bird flying into the sky – no footprints are left behind, not even a trace. The bird flies but leaves no path, no footprints.

The mind is just a process. In fact, mind doesn't exist, only thoughts – thoughts moving so fast that you think and feel that something exists there in continuity. One thought comes, another thought comes, another, and they go on. The gap between one thought and another is so small you cannot see it. So two thoughts become joined, they become a continuity, and because of that continuity you think there is a mind. There are thoughts – no mind; just as there are electrons – no matter. Thoughts are the electrons of the mind. Just like a crowd... A crowd exists in a sense, doesn't exist in another. Only individuals exist, but many individuals together give the feeling as if they are one. A nation exists and exists not; there are only individuals. Individuals are the electrons of a nation, of a community, of a crowd.

Thoughts exist, mind doesn't exist. Mind is just the appearance. And when you look deeper into the mind, it disappears. Then there are thoughts, but when the mind has disappeared and individual thoughts exist, many things are immediately solved. First thing: immediately you come to know that thoughts are like clouds. They come and go – and you are the sky. When there is no mind, immediately the perception comes that you are no longer involved in the thoughts. Thoughts are there, passing through you like clouds passing through the sky, or the wind passing through the trees. Thoughts are passing through you, and they can pass through because you are a vast emptiness. There is no hindrance, no obstacle. No wall exists to prevent them.

You are not a walled phenomenon. Your sky is infinitely open; thoughts come and go. And once you start feeling that thoughts come and go and you are the watcher, the witness, the mind is in control...

Osho
Yoga: The Mystery beyond Mind

introduction to the path of yoga

Now the discipline of Yoga.
Yoga is the cessation of mind.
Then the witness is established in itself.
In the other states there is identification
with the modifications of the mind.

We live in a deep illusion – an illusion of hope, of future, of tomorrow. As man is, he cannot exist without self-deception.

Nietzsche says somewhere that man cannot live with the true: he needs dreams, he needs illusions, he needs lies to exist. And Nietzsche is right. As man is he cannot exist with the truth. This has to be understood very deeply, because without understanding this, there can be no entry into the inquiry which is called Yoga.

The mind has to be understood deeply – the mind which needs lies, the mind which needs illusions, the mind which cannot exist with the real, the mind which needs dreams. You are not only dreaming in the night; even while awake you are continuously dreaming. You may be looking at me, you may be listening to me, but a dream current continuously goes on within you. The mind is creating dreams, images, fantasies.

Now scientists say that a man can live without sleep but he cannot live without dreams. In the old days it was understood that sleep was a necessity, but now modern research says sleep is not really a necessity; sleep is needed only so that you can dream. Dreaming is the necessity. If you are allowed to sleep but not allowed to dream, you will not feel fresh, alive, in the morning. You will feel tired, as if you have not been able to sleep at all.

In the night there are periods for deep sleep and periods for dreaming. There is a rhythm, just like day and night. There is a rhythm: in the beginning you fall into deep sleep for nearabout forty, forty-five minutes, then the dream phase comes in; then you dream; then again dreamless sleep, then again dreaming. This goes on the whole night. If your sleep is disturbed while you are deeply asleep without dreaming, when you wake in the morning you will not feel that you have missed anything. But if your dream is disturbed while you are dreaming, in the morning you will feel completely tired, exhausted.

Now this can be observed from the outside. If someone is sleeping you can judge whether he is dreaming or asleep. If he is dreaming his eyes will be continuously moving, as if he is seeing something with closed eyes. When he is fast asleep the eyes will not move; they will remain steady. So if your sleep is disturbed while your eyes are moving, in the morning you will feel tired. While your eyes are not moving sleep can be disturbed; in the morning you will not feel anything is missing.

Many researchers have proved that the human mind feeds on dreams; dreaming is a necessity, and dreaming is total auto-deception. And this is so not only in the night: while awake also the same pattern follows. Even in the day you can notice that sometimes there will be dreams floating in the mind, sometimes there will be no dreams.

When there are dreams you will be doing something but you will be absent. Inside you are occupied. For example, you are here. If your mind is passing through a dream-state you will listen to me without listening at all, because your mind will be occupied within. You can only listen to me if you are not in a dreaming state.

Day and night, mind goes on moving from no-dream to dream, then from dream to no-dream again. This is an inner rhythm. Not only do we continuously dream, in life also we project hopes into the future.

The present is almost always a hell: you can endure this hell only because of the hope that you have projected into the future. You can live today because of tomorrow. You are hoping something is going to happen tomorrow – the doors of paradise will open tomorrow. They never open today, and when tomorrow comes it will not come as tomorrow, it will come as today, but by that time your mind has moved again. You go on moving ahead of yourself: this is what dreaming means. You are not one with the real, that which is nearby, that which is here and now, you are somewhere else, moving ahead, jumping ahead.

You have named that tomorrow, that future, in many ways. Some people call it heaven, some people call it *moksha*, but it is always in the future. Somebody is thinking in terms of wealth, but that wealth is going to be in the future. And somebody is thinking in terms of paradise, and that paradise is going to be after you are dead, far away in the future. You waste your present for that which is not: this is what dreaming means. You cannot be here and now. To be just in the moment seems to be arduous.

You can be in the past, because again that is dreaming – memories, remembrance of things which are no more – or you can be in the future, which is projection, which again is creating something out of the past. The future is nothing but the past projected again. It may be more colorful, more beautiful, more pleasant, but it is the past refined.

You cannot think anything other than the past: the future is nothing but the past projected again. Future and past are not; the present is, but you are never in the present. This is what dreaming means. Nietzsche is right when he says that man cannot live with the truth. He needs lies, he lives through lies. Nietzsche says that we go on saying that we want the truth, but no one wants it. Our so-called truths are nothing but lies, beautiful lies. No one is ready to see the naked reality.

This mind cannot enter on the path of Yoga because Yoga is a methodology to reveal the truth. Yoga is a method to come to a non-dreaming mind. Yoga is the science to be in the here and now. Yoga means that now you are ready not to move into the future. Yoga means now you are ready not to hope, not to jump ahead of your being. Yoga means to encounter the reality as it is.

One can enter Yoga, or the path of Yoga, only when he is totally frustrated with his own mind as it is. If you are still hoping that you can

gain something through your mind, Yoga is not for you. A total frustration is needed – the revelation that the mind which projects is futile, the
mind that hopes is nonsense, it leads nowhere. It simply closes your
eyes, it intoxicates you, it never allows reality to be revealed to you. It
protects you against reality.

Your mind is a drug. It is against that which is. So you can enter
on the path only if you are totally frustrated with your mind, with your
way of being, with the way you have existed up to now, and you can
drop it unconditionally.

Many become interested but very few enter, because that interest
may be just because of the mind. You may be hoping that now,
through Yoga, you may gain something. The achieving motive is there
with the hope that you may become perfect through Yoga, you may
reach to the blissful state of perfect being, that you may become one
with the *brahman* that you may achieve the *satchitananda*. This may
be why you are interested in Yoga. If this is the cause then there can be
no meeting between you and the path which is Yoga. Then you are
totally against it, moving in a totally opposite dimension.

Yoga means: "Now no hope, now no future, now no desires. But
I am ready to know what is. I am not interested in what can be, what
should be, what ought to be. I am not interested! I am interested only
in that which is." Because only the real can free you, only the reality
can become liberation.

Total despair is needed. That despair Buddha called *dukkha*.
If you are really in misery don't hope, because your hope will only
prolong the misery. Your hope is a drug. It can help you to continue, but where are you moving? It will help you to reach only
death and nowhere else. All your hopes can lead you only to death;
they *are* leading.

Become totally hopeless – no future, no hope. It is difficult; it needs
courage to face the real. But such a moment comes to everyone,
sometime or other. A moment comes to every human being when he
feels total hopelessness. Absolute meaninglessness happens to him.
When he becomes aware that whatsoever he is doing is useless,
wheresoever he is going is going to nowhere, and all life is meaningless, then hopes drop. Future drops, and for the first time he is in tune
with the present, for the first time he is face to face with reality.

Unless this moment comes to you, you can go on doing *asanas,*
postures, but that is not Yoga. Yoga is an inward turning, a total

about-turn. When you are not moving into the future, not moving towards the past, then you start moving within yourself, because your being is here and now, it is not in the future. You are present here and now, you can enter this reality. But then mind has to be *here*.

This moment is indicated by the first sutra of Patanjali. Before we talk about the first sutra, a few other things have to be understood.

Yoga is not a religion, remember that. Yoga is not Hindu, it is not Mohammedan. Yoga is a pure science just like mathematics, physics or chemistry. Physics is not Christian, physics is not Buddhist. Christians may have discovered the laws of physics, but physics is not Christian. It is just accidental that Christians have come to discover the laws of physics. Physics remains just a science. Yoga is a science; it is just accidental that Hindus discovered it. It is not Hindu. It is pure mathematics of the inner being. A Mohammedan can be a yogi, a Christian can be a yogi, a Jaina, a Buddhist can be a yogi.

Yoga is pure science. And Patanjali is the greatest name in the world of Yoga. This man is rare; there is no other name comparable to Patanjali. For the first time in the history of humanity this man brought religion to the state of science. He made religion a science; a religion of pure laws, no belief is needed.

So-called religions need beliefs. There is no other difference between one religion and another except the difference of beliefs. A Mohammedan has certain beliefs, a Hindu certain others, a Christian certain others. The difference is of beliefs. Yoga has nothing as far as belief is concerned; Yoga doesn't say to believe in anything. Yoga says to experience. Just as science says to experience, Yoga says to experience. Experiment and experience are both the same; their directions are different. Experiment means there is something you can do outside; experience means there is something you can do inside. Experience is an inner experiment.

Science says, "Don't believe, doubt as much as you can," but also, "Don't disbelieve" – because disbelief is again a sort of belief. You can believe in God, you can believe in the concept of no-God. You can say that God exists with a fanatic attitude and you can say quite the reverse, that God exists not, with the same fanaticism. Atheists, theists, are all believers, and belief is not the realm of science. Science means to experience something, that which is; no belief is needed.

The second thing to remember is that Yoga is existential, experiential, experimental; no belief is required, no faith is needed. Only the courage to experience is needed, and that is what is lacking. You can believe easily because in belief you are not going to be transformed. Belief is something added to you, something superficial. Your being is not changed, you are not passing through some mutation. You may be a Hindu one day and become a Christian the next day, simply by changing the Gita for a Bible. You can change it for a Koran, but the man who was holding the Gita and is now holding the Bible remains the same; he has just changed his beliefs.

Beliefs are like clothes. Nothing substantial is transformed, you remain the same. Dissect a Hindu, dissect a Mohammedan – inside they are the same. The Hindu goes to a temple, the Mohammedan hates the temple. The Mohammedan goes to the mosque and the Hindu hates the mosque but inside they are the same human beings.

Belief is easy because you are not really required to do anything, just a superficial dressing, a decoration, something which you can put aside any moment you like. Yoga is not belief; that's why it is difficult, arduous, sometimes it seems impossible. It is an existential approach. You will come to the truth not through belief but through your own experience, through your own realization. That means you will have to be totally changed – your viewpoints, your way of life, your mind; your psyche as it is has to be shattered completely. Something new has to be created. Only with that new will you come in contact with the reality.

Yoga is both a death and a new life. As you are you will have to die, and unless you die the new cannot be born. The new is hidden in you. You are just a seed for it and the seed must fall down, be absorbed by the earth. The seed must die, only then will the new arise out of you. Your death will become your new life. Yoga is both a death and a new birth. Unless you are ready to die you cannot be reborn. So it is not a question of changing beliefs.

Yoga is not a philosophy. I say it is not a religion and I say it is not a philosophy. It is not something you can think about. It is something you will have to *be;* thinking won't do. Thinking goes on in your head. It is not really deep into the roots of your being, it is not your totality, it is just a part, a functional part. It can be trained and you can argue logically, you can think rationally, but your heart will remain the same. Your heart is your deepest center, your head is just a branch. You can be without the head but you cannot be without the heart. Your head is not basic.

Yoga is concerned with your total being, with your roots. It is not philosophical. So with Patanjali we will not be thinking, speculating. With Patanjali we will be trying to know the ultimate laws of being, the laws for its transformation, the laws of how to die and how to be reborn again, the laws for a new order of being. That is why I call it a science.

Patanjali is rare. He is an enlightened person like Buddha, like Krishna, like Christ, like Mahavira, Mohammed, Zarathustra, but he is different in one way. Buddha, Krishna, Mahavira, Zarathustra, Mohammed – none of them has a scientific attitude. They are great founders of religions. They have changed the whole pattern of the human mind and its structure, but their approach is not scientific.

Patanjali is like an Einstein in the world of buddhas. He is a phenomenon. He could easily have been a Nobel Prize winner like an Einstein or Bohr or Max Planck or Heisenberg. He has the same attitude, the same approach as a rigorous, scientific mind. He is not a poet; Krishna is a poet. He is not a moralist; Mahavira is a moralist. Patanjali is basically a scientist who is thinking in terms of laws. And he has come to deduce absolute laws of the human being, the ultimate working structure of the human mind and of reality.

If you follow Patanjali you will come to know that he is as exact as any mathematical formula. Simply do what he says and the result will happen. The result is bound to happen – it is just like two plus two equals four or like heating water to one hundred degrees causes it to evaporate. No belief is needed, you simply do it and know; it is something to be done and known. That's why I say there is no comparison: never has another man like Patanjali existed on this earth.

You can find poetry in Buddha's utterances; it is bound to be there. Many times while Buddha is expressing himself he becomes poetic. The realm of ecstasy, the realm of ultimate knowing is so beautiful, the temptation is strong to become poetic, the beauty is such, the benediction is such, the bliss is such that one starts talking in poetic language.

But Patanjali resists that. It is very difficult to resist, no one else has been able to. Jesus, Krishna, Buddha all became poetic. When the splendor, the beauty, explode within you, you will start dancing, you will start singing. In that state you are just like a lover who has fallen in love with the whole universe.

Patanjali resists that. He will not use poetry; he will not even use a single poetic symbol. He will not do anything with poetry. He will not talk in terms of beauty: he will talk in terms of mathematics, he will be exact. He will give you maxims, but those maxims are just indications of what is to be done. He will not explode into ecstasy, he will not say things that cannot be said, he will not try the impossible. He will just put down the foundation and if you follow the foundation you will reach the peak which is beyond. He is a rigorous mathematician, remember this.

The first sutra:

> Now the discipline of Yoga.
> Athayoganushasanam: Now the discipline of Yoga.

Each single word has to be understood, because Patanjali will not use a single superfluous word.

Now the discipline of Yoga. First try to understand the word now. This "now" is an indication to the state of mind I was just talking to you about.

If you are disillusioned, if you are hopeless, if you have completely become aware of the futility of all desires; if you see your life as meaningless; whatsoever you have been doing up to now has simply fallen dead, nothing remains in the future, you are in absolute despair – what Kierkegaard calls anguish – you are in anguish, suffering, not knowing what to do, not knowing where to go, not knowing to whom to turn, just on the verge of madness or suicide or death, your whole pattern of life has suddenly become futile; if this moment has come, Patanjali says: Now the discipline of Yoga – only now can you understand the science of Yoga, the discipline of Yoga.

If that moment has not come you can go on studying Yoga, and you can become a great scholar but you will not be a yogi. You can write theses on it, you can give discourses on it, but you will not be a yogi. The moment has not come for you. Intellectually you can become interested, through your mind you can be related to Yoga, but Yoga is nothing if it is not a discipline. Yoga is not a shastra; it is not a scripture. It is a discipline; it is something you have to do. It is not curiosity, it is not philosophical speculation, it is deeper than that. It is a question of life and death.

If the moment has come when you feel that all directions have become confused, all roads have disappeared, the future is dark and every desire has become bitter and through every desire you have known only disappointment, all movement into hopes and dreams has ceased: *Now the discipline of Yoga.*

This "now" may not have come. Then I may go on talking about Yoga but you will not listen. You can listen only if the moment is present in you. Are you really dissatisfied? Everybody will say yes, but that dissatisfaction is not real. You are dissatisfied with this, you may be dissatisfied with that, but you are not totally dissatisfied. You are still hoping. You are dissatisfied because of your past hopes but you are still hoping for the future. Your dissatisfaction is not total: you are still hankering for some satisfaction somewhere, for some gratification somewhere.

Sometimes you feel hopeless but that hopelessness is not true. You feel hopeless because certain hopes have not been achieved, certain hopes have fallen away, but hoping is still there, hoping has not fallen away. You will still hope. You are dissatisfied with this hope, that hope, but you are not dissatisfied with hope as such. If you are disappointed with hope as such the moment has come, and then you can enter Yoga. And then this entry will not be an entering into a mental, speculative phenomenon. This entry will be an entry into a discipline.

What is discipline? Discipline means creating an order within you. As you are, you are a chaos. As you are, you are totally disorderly. Gurdjieff used to say – and Gurdjieff is in many ways like Patanjali, he was again trying to make the core of religion a science – Gurdjieff said that you are not one, you are a crowd; not even when you say "I" is there any I. There are many I's in you, many egos. In the morning one I, in the afternoon another I, in the evening a third I, but you never become aware of this mess – because who will become aware of it? There is not a center that can become aware.

...the discipline of Yoga means Yoga wants to create a crystallized center in you. As you are, you are a crowd and a crowd has many phenomena. One is that you cannot believe a crowd. Gurdjieff used to say that man cannot promise: who will promise? You are not there. If you promise who will fulfill the promise? Next morning the one who promised is not there.

People come to me and they say, "Now I will take the vow. I promise to do this," and I tell them, "Think twice before you promise something. Are you confident that the next moment the one who promised it will be there?" You decide that starting tomorrow you will get up early in the morning at four o'clock, and at four o'clock somebody in you says, "Don't bother. It is so cold outside. And why are you in such a hurry? We can do it tomorrow" – and you fall asleep again. When you get up you repent and you think, "This is not good. I should have done it." You decide again, "Tomorrow I will do it"; and the same is going to happen tomorrow because at four in the morning the one who promised is no longer there, somebody else is in the chair. You are a Rotary Club: the chairman goes on changing and every member becomes a Rotary chairman. There is rotation: every moment someone else is the master.

Gurdjieff used to say, "This is the chief characteristic of man – that he cannot promise." You cannot fulfill a promise. You go on giving promises, and you know well that you cannot fulfill them because you are not one; you are a disorder, a chaos. Hence Patanjali says: *Now the discipline of Yoga.* If your life has become an absolute misery, if you have realized that whatsoever you do creates hell, then the moment has come. This moment can change your dimension, your direction of being.

Up until now you have lived as a chaos, a crowd. Yoga means now you will have to be a harmony, you will have to become one. A crystallization is needed, a centering is needed. And unless you attain a center all that you do is useless; it is wasting life and time. A center is the first necessity, and only a person who has a center can be blissful. Everybody asks for it, but you cannot ask for it, you have to earn it! Everybody hankers for a blissful state of being, but only a center can be blissful, a crowd cannot be blissful. A crowd has no self, there is no atman. Who is going to be blissful?

Bliss means absolute silence, and silence is possible only when there is harmony, when all the discordant fragments have become one, when there is no crowd, only one. When you are alone in the house and nobody else is there, you will be blissful. Right now everybody else is in your house, you are not there. Only the guests are there, the host is always absent, and only the host can be blissful.

This centering Patanjali calls discipline, *anushasanam.* The word *discipline* is beautiful. It comes from the same root as the word *disciple. Discipline* means the capacity to learn, the capacity to know. But you cannot know, you cannot learn unless you have attained the capacity to *be.*

A man once went to Buddha and he said – he must have been a social reformer, a revolutionary – he said to Buddha, "The world is in misery. I agree with you."

Buddha has never said that the world is in misery. Buddha says *you* are the misery, not the world; *life* is misery, not the world; *man* is misery, not the world; *mind* is misery, not the world. But that revolutionary said, "The world is in misery, I agree with you. Now tell me, what can I do? I have a deep compassion and I want to serve humanity."

Service must have been his motto! Buddha looked at him and remained silent. Buddha's disciple, Ananda, said, "This man seems to be sincere. Guide him. Why are you silent?"

Then Buddha said to that revolutionary, "You want to serve the world, but where are you? I don't see anyone inside. I look in you, and there is no one. You don't have any center, and unless you are centered whatsoever you do will create more mischief."

All your social reformers, your revolutionaries, your leaders, are the great mischief creators, mischief-mongers. The world would be better if there were no leaders. But they cannot help: they must do something because the world is in misery and they are not centered, so whatsoever they do will create more misery. Compassion alone will not help, service alone will not help. Compassion through a centered being is something totally different. Compassion through a crowd is mischief; that compassion is poison.

Now the discipline of Yoga.

Discipline means the capacity to be, the capacity to know, the capacity to learn. We must understand these three things.

The capacity to be... All the Yoga postures are not really concerned with the body, they are concerned with the capacity to be. Patanjali says if you can sit silently without moving your body for a few hours, you are growing in the capacity to be. Why do you move? You cannot sit without moving even for a few seconds: your body starts moving, somewhere you feel itching, the legs go dead, many things start happening – these are just excuses for you to move.

You are not a master. You cannot say to the body, "Now I will not move for one hour." The body will revolt immediately! Immediately it will force you to move, to do something. And it will give reasons: "You have to move because an insect is biting." You may not find the insect when you look. You are not a being, you are a trembling, a continuous hectic activity. Patanjali's *asanas*, postures, are not really concerned with any kind of physiological training but with an inner training of being: just to be, without doing anything, without any movement, without any activity. Just remain – that remaining will help centering.

If you can remain in one posture the body will become a slave; it will follow you. And the more the body follows you the more you will have a greater being within you, a stronger being within you. Remember, if the body is not moving your mind cannot move, because mind and body are not two things, they are two poles of one phenomenon. You are not body and mind, you are bodymind. Your personality is psychosomatic, bodymind, both. Mind is the most subtle part of the body, or you can say the reverse, that body is the grossest part of the mind. So whatsoever happens in the body happens in the mind and vice versa, whatsoever happens in the mind happens in the body. If the body is nonmoving and you can attain a posture, if you can say to the body, "Keep quiet," the mind will remain silent. Really, the mind starts moving and tries to move the body, because if the body moves then the mind can move. In a nonmoving body the mind cannot move; it needs a moving body.

If the body is nonmoving, the mind is nonmoving – you are centered. This nonmoving posture is not only a physiological training, it is to create a situation in which centering can happen, in which you can become disciplined. When you are, when you have become centered, when you know what it means to be, then you can learn because then you will be humble. Then you can surrender. Then no false ego will cling to you because once centered you know all egos are false. Then you can bow down. Then a disciple is born.

To become a disciple is a great achievement. Only through discipline will you become a disciple. Only through being centered will you become humble, will you become receptive, will you become empty and the guru, the master, can pour himself into you. In your emptiness, in your silence, he can come and reach to you. Communication becomes possible.

Disciple means one who is centered, humble, receptive, open, ready, alert, waiting, prayerful. In Yoga the master is very, very important, absolutely important, because only when you are in the close proximity of a being who is centered will your own centering happen.

That is the meaning of *satsang*. You have heard the word *satsang*; it is used totally wrongly. *Satsang* means, in close proximity to the truth; it means, near the truth, it means near a master who has become one with the truth – just being near him, open, receptive and waiting. If your waiting has become deep, intense, a deep communion will happen.

The master is not going to do anything. He is simply there, available. If you are open he will flow within you. This flowing is called *satsang*. With a master you need not learn anything else. If you can learn *satsang*, that's enough. If you can just be near him without asking, without thinking, without arguing; just present there, available, so the being of the master can flow in you, it is enough. And being can flow; it is already flowing. Whenever a person achieves integrity his being becomes a radiation. He is flowing. Whether you are there to receive or not is not the point. He flows like a river, and if you are empty like a vessel, ready, open, he will flow in you.

A disciple is one who is ready to receive, who has become a womb; the master can penetrate into him. This is the meaning of the word *satsang*. It is not basically a discourse; *satsang* is not a discourse. There may be a discourse but the discourse is just an excuse. You are here and I will talk on Patanjali's sutras, but that is just an excuse. If you are really here then the discourse, the talk, becomes just an excuse for your being here, for you to be here. And if you are *really* here, *satsang* starts. I can flow, and that flow is deeper than any talk, any communication through language, than any intellectual meeting with you.

If you are a disciple, if you are a disciplined being, if your mind is engaged in listening to me, then your being can be in *satsang*. Then your head is occupied. If your heart is open then on a deeper level a meeting happens. That meeting is *satsang*, and everything else is just an excuse to find ways to be close to the master.

Closeness is all, but only a disciple can be close. Anybody and everybody cannot be close. Closeness means a loving trust. Why are we not close? – because there is fear. Too close may be dangerous, too open may be dangerous, because you become vulnerable and then it will be difficult for you to defend. So just as a security measure we keep everybody at a distance, we never allow anyone to enter a certain space.

Everybody has a territory around him. Whenever somebody enters your territory you become afraid. Everybody has a space to protect. You are sitting alone in your room and a stranger enters into the room: just watch when you become really scared. There is a point that if he enters that point you will become scared, you will be afraid. A sudden trembling will be felt. He cannot move beyond a certain territory.

To be close means that now you have no territory of your own. To be close means to be vulnerable; to be close means that whatsoever happens, you are not thinking in terms of security.

A disciple can be close for two reasons. One: he is centered or he is trying to be centered. A person who is even trying to be centered becomes unafraid; he becomes fearless. He has something which cannot be killed. You don't have anything, hence the fear. You are a crowd. The crowd can disperse at any moment. You don't have something like a rock which will be there whatsoever happens. You are existing without a rock, without a foundation; a house of cards, bound to be always in fear. Any wind, even any breeze can destroy you, so you have to protect yourself.

Because of this constant protection you cannot love, you cannot trust, you cannot be friendly. You may have many friends but there is no friendship, because friendship needs closeness. You may have wives and husbands and so-called lovers but there is no love because love needs closeness, love needs trust. You may have gurus, masters but there is no disciplehood, because you cannot allow yourself to be totally given to somebody's being; nearness to his being, closeness to his being, so he can overpower you, flood over you.

A disciple is a seeker who is not a crowd, who is trying to be centered and crystallized, who is at least trying, making efforts, sincere efforts to become individual, to feel his being, to become his own master. The whole discipline of Yoga is an effort to make you a master of yourself. As you are, you are just a slave of many, many desires. Many, many masters are there and you are just a slave pulled in many directions.

Now the discipline of Yoga.

Yoga is discipline. It is an effort on your part to change yourself. Many other things have to be understood. Yoga is not a therapy. In the West many psychological therapies are now prevalent, and many Western psychologists think that Yoga is also a therapy. It is not; it is a discipline. What is the difference? This is the difference: a therapy is needed if you are ill, a therapy is needed if you are diseased, a therapy is needed if you are pathological. A discipline is needed even when you are healthy. Really, only when you are healthy can a discipline help; it is not for pathological cases.

Yoga is for those who are completely healthy as far as medical science is concerned, normal. They are not schizophrenic, they are not mad, they are not neurotic. They are normal people, healthy people with no particular pathology. Still they become aware that whatsoever is called normality is futile, whatsoever is called health is of no use. Something more is needed, something greater is needed; something holier and whole is needed.

Therapies are for ill people. Therapies can help you to come to Yoga, but Yoga is not a therapy. Yoga is for a higher order of health, a different order of health, a different type of being and wholeness. Therapy can, at the most, make you adjusted. Freud says we cannot do more. We can make you an adjusted, normal member of the society, but if the society itself is pathological, then what? And it is! The society itself is ill. A therapy can make you normal in the sense that you are adjusted to the society, but the society itself is ill.

So sometimes it happens that in an ill society a healthy person is thought to be ill. A Jesus is thought to be ill and every effort is done to make him adjusted. And when it is found that he is a hopeless case then he is crucified. When it is found that nothing can be done, that this man is incurable, then he is crucified. The society is itself ill because society is nothing but a collective. If all the members are ill the society is ill, and every member has to be adjusted to it.

Yoga is not therapy; Yoga is not trying in any way to make you adjusted to the society. If you want to define Yoga in terms of adjustment then it is not adjustment with the society, but it is adjustment with existence itself. It is adjustment with the divine.

So it may happen that a perfect yogi may appear mad to you. He may look out of his senses, out of his mind, because now he is in touch with the greater, with a higher mind, a higher order of things. He is in touch with the universal mind. It has always happened so:

a Buddha, a Jesus, a Krishna always looks somehow eccentric. They don't belong to us, they seem to be outsiders.

That's why they call them *avataras,* outsiders. They have come as if from some other planet, they don't belong to us. They may be higher, they may be good, they may be divine, but they don't belong to us. They come from somewhere else. They are not part and parcel of our being, mankind. The feeling has persisted that they are outsiders. They are not; they are the *real* insiders because they have touched the inner-most core of existence. But to us they appear outsiders.

Now the discipline of Yoga.

If your mind has come to realize that whatsoever you have been doing up to now was just senseless, it was a nightmare at the worst or a beautiful dream at the best, then the path of discipline opens before you. What is that path? The basic definition is:

Yoga is the cessation of mind – chittavrittinirodha.

I told you that Patanjali is mathematical. In a single sentence: *Now the discipline of Yoga,* he is finished with *you.* This is the only sentence that has been used for you. Now he takes it for granted that you are interested in Yoga not as a hope but as a discipline, as a transformation right here and now. He proceeds to define:

Yoga is the cessation of mind.

This is the definition of Yoga, the best definition. Yoga has been defined in many ways; there are many definitions. Some say Yoga is the meeting of the mind with the divine; hence, it is called Yoga – *Yoga* means meeting, joining together. Some say that Yoga means dropping the ego, ego is the barrier: the moment you drop the ego you are joined to the divine. You were already joined; it only appeared that you were not joined because of the ego. There are many definitions, but Patanjali's is the most scientific. He says: *Yoga is the cessation of mind.*

Yoga is the state of no-mind. The word *mind* covers everything – your egos, your desires, your hopes, your philosophies, your reli-gions, your scriptures. *Mind* covers all. Whatsoever you can think is mind. All that is known, all that can be known, all that is knowable, is within mind. Cessation of the mind means cessation of the known, cessation of the knowable. It is a jump into the unknown. When there is no-mind you are in the unknown. Yoga is a jump into the unknown. It will not be right to say "unknown"; rather, "unknowable."

What is the mind? What is the mind doing there? What is it? Ordinarily we think that mind is something substantial there, inside the head. Patanjali doesn't agree, and no one who has ever known the inside of the mind will agree. Modern science also doesn't agree. Mind is not something substantial inside the head. Mind is just a function, just an activity.

You walk, and I say you are walking. What is walking? If you stop, where is walking? If you sit down, where has the walking gone? Walking is nothing substantial; it is an activity. So while you are sitting no one can ask, "Where have you put your walking? Just now you were walking, so where has the walking gone?" You will laugh. You will say, "Walking is not something substantial, it is just an activity. I can walk. I can again walk and I can stop. It is activity."

Mind is also activity, but because of the word *mind* it appears as if something substantial is there. It is better to call it "minding" – just like walking. Mind means "minding," mind means thinking. It is an activity.

Again and again I have been quoting Bodhidharma...

Bodhidharma went to China and the emperor of China came to see him. The emperor said, "My mind is very uneasy, very disturbed. You are a great sage and I have been waiting for you. Tell me what I should do to put my mind at peace."

Bodhidharma said, "Don't do anything. First, bring your mind to me."

The emperor could not follow. He said, "What do you mean?"

He said, "Come in the morning at four o'clock, when nobody is here. Come alone, and remember to bring your mind with you."

The emperor couldn't sleep the whole night. Many times he canceled the whole idea: "This man seems to be mad. What does he mean, 'Come with your mind, don't forget'?" But the man was so enchanting, so charismatic that the emperor couldn't cancel the appointment. As if a magnet were pulling him, at four o'clock he jumped out of the bed and said, "Whatsoever happens, I must go.

This man may have something; his eyes say that he has something. He looks a little crazy, but still I must go and see what can happen."

So he arrived, and Bodhidharma was sitting with his big staff. And he said, "So you have come? Where is your mind? Have you brought it or not?"

The emperor said, "You talk nonsense. When I am here my mind is here, and it is not something which I can forget somewhere. It is in me."

So Bodhidharma said, "Okay. So the first thing is decided – that the mind is within you."

The emperor said, "Okay, the mind is within me."

Bodhidharma said, "Now close your eyes and find out where it is. And if you can find out where it is, immediately indicate to me. I will put it at peace."

So the emperor closed his eyes, tried and tried, looked and looked. The more he looked the more he became aware that there is no mind, that mind is an activity. It is not something there so you can pinpoint it. But the moment he realized that it is not something, then the absurdity of his quest became exposed to him: "If it is not something, nothing can be done about it. If it is an activity, then don't do the activity; that's all. If it is like walking, don't walk."

He opened his eyes. He bowed down to Bodhidharma and said, "There is no mind to be found."

Bodhidharma said, "Then I have put it at peace. And whenever you feel that you are uneasy, just look within for where that uneasiness is."

The very looking is anti-mind, because a look is not a thinking. And if you look intensely your whole energy becomes a look, and the same energy becomes movement and thinking.

Yoga is the cessation of mind.

This is Patanjali's definition: when there is no mind you are in Yoga, when there is mind you are not in Yoga. So you may do all the postures but if the mind goes on functioning, if you go on thinking, you are not in Yoga.

Yoga is the state of no-mind. If you can be without the mind without doing any posture, you have become a perfect yogi. It has happened to many without doing any postures, and it has not happened to many who have been doing postures for many lives. Because the basic thing to be understood is: when the activity of thinking is not there, *you* are there. When the activity of the mind is not there, when thoughts have disappeared – they are just like clouds – when they have disappeared your being, just like the sky, is uncovered. It is always there, only covered with the clouds, only covered with thoughts.

Yoga is the cessation of mind.

Now in the West there is much appeal for Zen which is a Japanese method of Yoga. The word *Zen* comes from *dhyana*. Bodhidharma introduced this word *dhyana* into China. The word *dhyana* became *jhan,* and then in China *ch'an,* and then the word traveled to Japan and became *Zen.*

The root is *dhyana. Dhyana* means no-mind, so the whole training of Zen in Japan is nothing but how to stop "minding," how to be a no-mind, how to be simply without thinking. Try it! When I say try it, it will look contradictory, but there is no other way to say it, because if you try, the very trying, the effort, is coming from the mind. You can sit in a posture and you can try some *japa*, chanting a mantra, or you can just try to sit silently, not to think. But then "not to think" becomes the thinking. Then you go on saying, "I am not to think, don't think, stop thinking," but this is all thinking.

Try to understand. When Patanjali says no-mind …*cessation of mind,* he means complete cessation. He will not allow you to make a mantra, "Ram-Ram-Ram." He will say that this is not cessation, you are using the mind. He will say, "Simply stop!" But you will ask, "How? How can you simply stop?" The mind continues. Even if you sit the mind continues. Even if you don't do, it goes on doing.

Patanjali says, "Then just look. Let mind go, let mind do whatsoever it is doing. You just look. You don't interfere. You just be a witness. You just be an onlooker, not concerned, as if the mind doesn't belong to you, as if it is not your business, not your concern. Don't be concerned. Just look and let the mind flow. It is flowing because of past momentum, because you have always helped it to flow. The activity has taken its own momentum, so it is flowing. Just don't cooperate. Look, and let the mind flow."

For many, many lives, perhaps a million lives, you have cooperated with it, you have helped it, you have given your energy to it. The river will flow for a while. If you don't cooperate, if you just look, unconcerned – Buddha's word is *indifference, upeksha:* looking without any concern, just looking, not doing anything in any way – the mind will flow for a while and it will stop by itself. When the momentum is lost, when the energy has flowed, the mind will stop. When the mind stops you are in Yoga: you have attained the discipline. This is the definition:

> *Yoga is the cessation of mind.*
> *Then the witness is established in itself.*

When the mind ceases ...*the witness is established in itself.*

When you can simply look without being identified with the mind, without judging, without appreciating, condemning, without choosing; you simply look and the mind flows, a time comes when by itself, of itself, the mind stops.

When there is no-mind you are established in your witnessing. Then you have become a witness, just a seer, a *drashta,* a *sakshi.* Then you are not a doer, then you are not a thinker. Then you are simply being, pure being, purest of being. *Then the witness is established in itself.*

> *In the other states there is identification*
> *with the modifications of the mind.*

Except witnessing, in all states you are identified with the mind. You become one with the flow of thoughts, you become one with the clouds: sometimes with the white cloud, sometimes with the black cloud, sometimes with a rain-filled cloud, sometimes with a vacant, empty cloud. But when you become one with the thought, you become one with the cloud, and you miss the purity of the sky, the purity of the space. You become clouded and this clouding happens because you get identified, you become one.

A thought comes. You are hungry and the thought flashes in the mind. The thought is simply that there is hunger, the stomach is feeling hunger. Immediately you get identified; you say, "*I* am hungry." The mind was just filled with a thought that hunger is

there, and you have become identified and you say, "*I* am hungry."
This is identification.

Buddha also feels hunger, Patanjali also feels hunger, but Patanjali
will never say, "I am hungry": he will say, "The body is hungry";
he will say, "My stomach is feeling hungry"; he will say, "There is
hunger. I am a witness. I have come to witness this thought which has
been flashed by the belly into the brain: 'I am hungry.'" The belly is
hungry, Patanjali will remain a witness. You become identified, you
become one with the thought.

> *Then the witness is established in itself.*
> *In the other states there is identification*
> *with the modifications of the mind.*

This is the definition:

> *Yoga is the cessation of mind.*

When mind ceases you are established in your witnessing self. In
other states except this there are identifications. And all identifications constitute the *sansar;* they are the world. If you are in the identifications you are in the world, in the misery. If you have transcended
the identifications you are liberated. You have become a *siddha,* you
are in nirvana. You have transcended this world of misery and
entered the world of bliss.

And that world is here and now – right now, this very moment!
You need not wait for even a single moment. Just become a witness
of the mind and you have entered. Get identified with the mind and
you have missed. This is the basic definition.

Remember everything, because later on, in other sutras, we will
go into details about what is to be done, how it is to be done.

But always keep in mind that this is the foundation: one has to
achieve a state of no-mind. That is the goal.

Enough for today.

desireless, you are enlightened

The first question:

Osho,
You said last night that total despair, frustration and
hopelessness is the beginning ground for Yoga. This
gives Yoga a pessimistic look. Is this pessimistic state
really necessary to begin the path of Yoga? Can an
optimist also begin with the path of Yoga?

It is neither pessimistic nor optimistic, because pessimism and
optimism are two aspects of the same coin. A pessimist is one
who was an optimist in the past; an optimist is one who will be a
pessimist in the future. All optimism leads to pessimism because
every hope leads to hopelessness.

If you are still hoping then Yoga is not for you. The desire is there,
hope is there; *sansar*, the world is there. Your desire is the world, your
hope is the bondage, because hope will not allow you to be in the
present. It will go on forcing you towards the future; it will not allow
you to be centered. It will pull and push but it will not allow you to
remain in a restful moment, in a state of stillness. It will not allow you.

So when I say total hopelessness I mean that hope has failed and hopelessness has also become futile. Then it is total hopelessness. Total hopelessness means even hopelessness is not there, because when you feel hopeless a subtle hope is there. Otherwise why should you feel hopeless? Hope is there, you are still clinging to it; hence the hopelessness.

Total hopelessness means now there is no hope. And when there is no hope there cannot be hopelessness. You have simply dropped the whole phenomenon. Both aspects have been thrown out, the whole coin has been dropped. In this state of mind you can enter the path of Yoga, never before. Before there is no possibility: hope is against Yoga.

Yoga is not pessimistic. You may be optimistic or pessimistic; Yoga is neither. If you are pessimistic you cannot enter on the path of Yoga because a pessimist clings to his miseries. He will not allow his miseries to disappear. An optimist clings to his hopes and a pessimist clings to his miseries, to his hopelessness. That hopelessness has become the companion. Yoga is for the one who is neither, who has become so totally hopeless that even to feel hopelessness is futile.

The opposite can be felt only if you go on clinging with the positive somewhere deep down. If you cling to hope you can feel hopelessness. If you cling to expectation you can feel frustration. If you simply come to realize that there is no possibility of expecting anything, then where is the frustration? Then this is the nature of existence, that there is no possibility of expecting anything, there is no possibility of hope. When this becomes a certainty, how can you feel hopeless? Then both have disappeared.

Patanjali says: *Now the discipline of Yoga.* That *now* will happen only when you are neither positive nor negative. Both pessimistic attitudes and optimistic attitudes are ill. But there are teachers who go on talking in terms of optimism, particularly American Christian missionaries. They go on talking in terms of hope, optimism, future, heaven. In the eyes of Patanjali that is just juvenile, childish, because you are simply giving a new disease. You are substituting a new disease for the old. You are unhappy and somehow you are seeking happiness. So whosoever gives you an assurance that, "This is the path that will lead you to happiness," you will follow it. He is giving you hope, but the misery you are feeling so much is because of your past hopes; he is simply creating a future hell.

Yoga expects you to be more adult, more mature. Yoga says there is no possibility to expect anything; there is no possibility of any fulfillment in the future. There is no heaven in the future waiting for you and no God waiting for you with Christmas gifts. There is nobody waiting for you so don't hanker after the future.

When you become aware that there is nothing which is going to happen somewhere in the future, you will become alert here and now because there is nowhere to move. Then there is no way to tremble, a stillness happens to you. Suddenly you are in a deep rest. You cannot go anywhere; you are at home. Movement ceases, restlessness disappears. Now is the time to enter Yoga.

Patanjali will not give you any hope. He respects you more than you respect yourself. He thinks you are mature and toys will not help. It is better to be alert to whatever is the case. But immediately when I say, "Total hopelessness" your mind will say, "This appears pessimistic," because your mind lives through hope, your mind clings to desires, expectations.

You are so miserable right now that you will commit suicide if there is no hope. Really, if Patanjali is true, what will happen to you? If there is no hope, no future and you are thrown back to your present, you will commit suicide. Then there is nothing to live for. You live for something which will happen somewhere, sometime. It is not going to happen, but the feeling that it may happen helps you to stay alive.

That's why I say when you have come to a point where suicide has become a meaningful thing, where life has lost all its meaning, where you can kill yourself, in that moment Yoga becomes possible because you will not be ready to transform yourself unless this intense futility of life has happened to you. You will be ready to transform yourself only when you feel there is no way except suicide or sadhana, either commit suicide or transform your being. When only two alternatives are left, only then is Yoga chosen, never before. But Yoga is not pessimistic. You are optimistic so Yoga appears to you as pessimistic. It is because of you.

In the West Buddha has been taken as the peak of pessimism because Buddha says life is dukkha, anguish. Therefore Western philosophers have been commenting that Buddha is a pessimist. Even a person like Albert Schweitzer, a person we can expect to know certain things, even he is in confusion. He thinks the whole East is pessimistic and this is a great criticism for him. The whole East – Buddha, Patanjali, Mahavira, Lao Tzu, are all pessimists for him. They do appear so; they appear so because they say your life is meaningless. Not that they say life is meaningless, but the life that *you* know. And unless this life becomes absolutely meaningless you cannot transcend it, you will cling to it.

Unless you transcend this life, this mode of existence, you will not know what bliss is. But Buddha or Patanjali will not talk much about bliss because they have a deep compassion for you. If they start talking about bliss you again create a hope. You are incurable: you again create a hope. You say, "Okay! Then we can leave this life. If a more abundant life, a richer life is possible, then we can leave desires. If through leaving desires the deepest desire of reaching to the ultimate, the peak of bliss, is possible, then we can leave desires. But we can leave only for a greater desire."

Then where are you leaving? You are not leaving at all. You are simply substituting a different desire for the old one. And the new desire will be more dangerous than the old because you are already frustrated with the old. To get frustrated with the new you may again take even a few lives to come to a point where you can say God is useless, where you can say heaven is foolish, where you can say all future is nonsense.

It is not a question of worldly desires; it is a question of desire *as such*. Desiring must cease. Only then you become ready, only then you gather courage, only then the door opens and you can enter into the unknown. Hence, Patanjali's first sutra: *Now the discipline of Yoga.*

The second question:

Osho,
It is said that Yoga is an atheistic system. Do you agree with this?

Again, Yoga is neither. It is a simple science. It is neither theistic nor atheistic. Patanjali really is superb, a miracle of a man. He never talks about God. And even if he mentions God once, then too he says it is just one of the methods of reaching the ultimate. The belief in God is just a method to reach the ultimate – there is no God. To believe in God is just a technique, because through believing in God prayerfulness becomes possible; through believing in God surrender becomes possible. The significance is of surrender and prayerfulness, not of God.

Patanjali is really unbelievable! He said God – the belief in God, the concept of God – is also one of the methods among many methods to reach the truth. *Ishwara pranidhan* – to believe in God is just a path. But it is not a necessity. You can choose something else. Buddha reaches to that ultimate reality without believing in God. He chooses a different path where God is not needed.

You have come to my house, you have passed through a certain street, but that street was not the goal, it was just instrumental. You could have reached to the same house through some other street; others have reached through other streets. On your street there may be green trees, big trees, on other streets there may not be. So God is just one path. Remember the distinction: God is not the goal. God is just one of the paths.

Patanjali never denies, he never assumes. He is absolutely scientific. It is difficult for Christians to understand how Buddha could attain the ultimate truth, because he never believed in God. It is difficult for Hindus to understand how Mahavira could attain liberation, because he never believed in God.

Before the Western thinkers became alert about Eastern religions they always defined religion as God-centered. When they came upon Eastern thinking and they became aware that there has been a traditional path, a godless path reaching toward truth, they were shocked: "It is impossible!"

H. G. Wells has written about Buddha that Buddha is the most godless man and yet the most godly. He never believed and he will never tell anybody to believe in any God, but he himself is the suprememost phenomenon of the happening of divine being. Mahavira too travels a path where God is not needed.

Patanjali is absolutely scientific: he says we are not related with means, there are a thousand and one means – the goal is the truth. Some have achieved it through God, so it is okay – believe in God and achieve the goal, because when the goal is achieved you will throw away your belief. So belief is just instrumental. If you don't believe it is okay, don't believe, and travel the path of belieflessness and reach the goal.

He is neither theist nor atheist. He is not creating a religion, he is simply showing you all the paths that are possible and all the laws that work in your transformation. God is one of those paths, it is not a must. If you are godless there is no need to be non-religious. Patanjali says you can also reach, so be godless, don't bother about God. These are the laws and these are the experiments; this is the meditation – pass through it.

He does not insist on any concept. It was very difficult. That's why the *Yoga Sutras* of Patanjali are rare, unique. Such a book has never happened before and there is no possibility of its happening again, because whatsoever can be written about Yoga he has written, he has left nothing out. No one can add anything to it. Never in the future is there any possibility to create another work like Patanjali's *Yoga Sutras*. He has finished the job completely, and he could do this so totally because he is not partial. If he were partial then he could not do it so totally.

Buddha is partial, Mahavira is partial, Jesus is partial, Mohammed is partial – they have a certain path. And their partiality may be because of you, because of a deep compassion for you. They insist on a certain path, they go on insisting their whole life. And they say, "Everything else is wrong, this is the right path," just to create faith in you. You are so faithless; you are so filled with doubt that if they say, "This path leads, others' paths also lead," you will not follow any. They insist that only *this* path leads.

This is not true. This is just a device for you because if you feel any uncertainty in them, if they say, "This also leads, that also leads; this is also true, that is also true," you will become uncertain. You are already uncertain. You need someone who is absolutely certain. Just to look certain to you they have pretended to be partial.

But if you are partial you cannot cover the whole ground. Patanjali is not partial. He is less concerned with you, more concerned with the past designs of the path. He will not use a lie; he will not use a device, he will not compromise with you. No scientist can compromise.

Buddha can compromise. He has compassion, he is not treating you scientifically. A very deep human feeling is there for you; he can even lie just to help you. You cannot understand the truth so he compromises with you.

Patanjali will not compromise with you. Whatsoever is the fact, he will talk about the fact. And he will not descend a single step to meet you, he is absolutely uncompromising. Science has to be. Science cannot compromise; otherwise it will itself become a religion. He is neither atheist nor theist. He is neither Hindu nor Mohammedan nor Christian nor Jaina nor Buddhist. He is absolutely a scientific seeker just revealing whatsoever is the case, revealing without any myth. He will not use a single parable. Jesus will talk in stories because you are children and you can only understand stories. He will talk in parables. Buddha uses many stories just to help you to attain a little glimpse.

I was reading about a Hassid, a Jewish master, Baal Shem. He was a rabbi in a small village, and whenever there was some trouble, some disease, some calamity in the village, he would move into the forest. He would go to a certain spot under a certain tree and there he would do some ritual and then he would pray to God. And it always happened that the calamity would leave the village, the illness would disappear from the village, the trouble would go.

Then Baal Shem died. His successor came. Then a problem arose again, the village was in trouble. There was some calamity and the villagers asked the successor, the new rabbi, to go to the forest and pray to God. The new rabbi was very much disturbed because he was unacquainted with the spot, the exact tree. But still he went, stopped under any tree. He burned the fire, did the ritual and prayed and said to God, "Look, I don't know the exact spot my master used to come to, but you know. You are omnipotent, you are omnipresent, so you know, so there is no need to seek for the exact spot. My village is in some trouble, so listen and do something." The calamity was gone.

Then when this rabbi died and his successor was there, again the problem came. The village was in a certain crisis and they came to him. The rabbi was disturbed, he had even forgotten the prayer. So he went into the forest, chose any place. He didn't know how to burn the ritual fire but anyhow he burned a fire and said to God, "Listen, I don't know how to burn the ritual fire, I don't know the exact spot and I have forgotten the prayer. But you are all-knowing so you know already; there is no need for me to know. So do whatsoever is needed." And he came back and the village passed through the crisis.

Then he also died. Again the successor... And again the village was in trouble, so they came. He was sitting in his armchair. He said to God, "I don't want to go anywhere. Listen, you are everywhere.

I don't know the prayer, I don't know any ritual. But that doesn't matter; my knowing is not the point. You know everything. What is the use of praying and what is the use of a ritual and what is the use of a particular sacred spot? I know only the story of my successors. I will tell you the story that happened in Baal Shem's time, then his successor, then his successor: this is the story. Now do the right thing and this is enough." And the calamity disappeared. It is said that God loved the story so much.

People love their stories, and the people's God also loves stories, and through stories you can have certain glimpses. But Patanjali will not use a single parable. I told you he is just Einstein plus Buddha, a very rare combination. He has the inner witnessing of Buddha and the mechanism of mind of an Einstein, but he is neither.

Theism is a story, atheism is the anti-story. They are just myths, man-created parables. To some the one appeals, to some the other. Patanjali is not interested in stories or myths, he is interested in the naked truth. He will not even clothe it, he will not put on any dressing, he will not decorate it. That is not his way, remember this.

We will move on a very dry land, a desert-like land. But the desert has its own beauty. It has no trees, it has no rivers, but it has a vastness of its own. No forest can be compared to it. Forests have their own beauty, hills have their own beauty, rivers their own beauty. The desert has its own vast infinity.

We will be moving through desert-land. Courage is needed. He will not give you a single tree to rest under. He will not give you any story, just the bare facts. He will not use even a single superfluous word; hence the word *sutra*. *Sutra* means the basic minimum.

A sutra is not even a complete sentence. It is just the essential, just as when you write a telegram you cut out superfluous words. Then it becomes a sutra because only ten words or nine words can be put in it. If you were going to write a letter you would fill ten pages, and even in ten pages the message would not be complete. But in a telegram in ten words it is not only complete, it is more than complete. It hits the heart, the very essence is there.

Patanjali's sutras are telegrams. He is a miser, he will not use a single superfluous word. So how can he tell stories? – he cannot. And don't expect it. So don't ask whether he is a theist or an atheist; those are stories.

Philosophers have created many stories, and it is a game. If you like the game of atheism, be an atheist. If you like the game of theism, be a theist. But these are games, not the reality. Reality is something else. Reality is concerned with you, not what you believe. The reality *is* you, not what you believe. The reality is behind the mind, not in the contents of the mind. Because theism is a content of the mind, atheism is a content of the mind, something in the mind. Hinduism is a content of the mind or Christianity is a content of the mind.

Patanjali is concerned with the beyond, not with the content. He says, "Throw out this whole mind. Whatsoever it contains, it is useless." You may be carrying beautiful philosophies; Patanjali will say, "Throw them out! All is rubbish." It is difficult. If someone says, "Your Bible is rubbish, your Gita is rubbish, your scriptures are rubbish, rot, throw them away," you will be shocked. But this is how it is going to happen. Patanjali cannot make any compromise with you. He is uncompromising and that's the beauty. And that is his uniqueness.

The third question:

Osho,
You talked about the significance of discipleship on the path of Yoga, but how can an atheist be a disciple?

Neither a theist nor an atheist can be a disciple. They have already taken an attitude, they have already decided, so what is the point of being a disciple? If you already know how can you be a disciple? Discipleship means the realization that, "I don't know." Atheists, theists – no, they cannot be disciples.

And if you believe in something you will miss the beauty of disciplehood. If you know something already, that knowing will give you ego; it will not make you humble. That's why pundits and scholars miss. Sometimes sinners have reached, but scholars never. They know too much, they are so clever. Their cleverness is the disease that becomes their suicide. They won't listen because they are not ready to learn.

Disciplehood simply means an attitude to learn, a moment-to-moment remaining aware that "I don't know." This knowing that "I don't know," this awareness that "I am ignorant" gives you opening.

Then you are not closed. The moment you say "I know" you are a closed circle; the door is no longer open. But when you say "I don't know" it means you are ready to learn, the door is open.

If you have already reached, concluded, you cannot be a disciple. One has to be in a receptive mood. One has to be completely aware that the real is unknown, "And whatsoever I know is trivial, is just rubbish." What do you know? You may have gathered much information but that is not knowledge. You may have accumulated much dust through universities; that is not knowledge. You may know about Buddha, you may know about Jesus, but that is not knowledge. Unless you become a Buddha there is no knowledge. Unless you are a Jesus there is no knowledge.

Knowledge comes through being, not through memory. You can have a trained memory; memory is just a mechanism. It will not give you a richer being. It may give you nightmarish dreams but it will not give you a richer being. You will remain the same, covered with much dust. Knowledge, and particularly the ego that comes through knowledge – the feeling that "I know" – closes you. Now you cannot be a disciple. And if you cannot be a disciple you cannot enter the discipline of Yoga. So come to the door of Yoga ignorant, aware of your ignorance, alert that you don't know. And I will tell you: this is the only knowledge which will help, the knowledge that "I don't know."

This will make you humble. A subtle humility will come to you. The ego, by and by, will subside. Knowing that you don't know, how can you be egoistic? Knowledge is the most subtle food for the ego: you feel you are something. You know, therefore you become somebody.

Just two days ago I initiated a girl from the West into sannyas and I gave her a name, Yoga Sambodhi, and I asked her, "Will it be easy for you to pronounce?" She said, "Yes. It looks just like the English word *somebody*." But *sambodhi* is quite the opposite. When you become nobody, then *sambodhi* happens. *Sambodhi* means enlightenment. If you are somebody, *sambodhi* will never happen. That "somebodiness" is the barrier.

When you feel you are nobody, when you feel you are nothing, suddenly you are available for many mysteries to happen to you. Your doors are open. The sun can rise, the sunrays can penetrate you. Your gloom, your darkness, will disappear. But you are closed.

The sun may be knocking on the door but there is no opening, not even a window is open.

Atheists or theists, Hindus or Mohammedans, Christians or Buddhists, cannot enter on the path. They believe they have already reached Buddha without reaching anywhere. They have concluded without any realization. They have words in the mind, concepts, theories, scriptures – and the more the burden, the more dead they are.

The fourth question:

Osho,
You said that Yoga does not ask for any faith. But if a disciple needs faith, surrender and trust in the master as a basic condition, then how is the first statement valid?

I did not say that Yoga doesn't ask for faith. I said Yoga doesn't ask for any *belief*. Faith is totally different, trust is totally different. Belief is an intellectual thing, but faith is a very deep intimacy, it is not intellectual. You love a master, then you trust and there is faith. But this faith is not in any concept, it is in the very person. And this is not a condition, it is not required. Remember this distinction: it is not required that you must have faith in the master, it is not a precondition. All that is said is this: if trust happens between you and the master, then *satsang* will be possible. It is just a situation, not a condition. Nothing is required.

Just as with love: if love happens then marriage can follow, but you cannot make love a condition that first you must love and then marriage will follow. But then you will ask, "How can one love?" If it happens it happens, if it is not happening it is not happening. You cannot do anything. So you cannot force trust.

In the old days seekers would roam all over the world. They would roam from one master to another, just waiting for the phenomenon to happen. You cannot force it. You may pass through many masters just in a search to see if somewhere something clicks. Then the thing has happened; it is not a condition. You cannot go to a master and try to trust him. How can you try to trust? The very trying, the very effort shows you don't trust. How can you try to love someone? If you try, the whole thing has become false. It is a happening.

But unless this happens, *satsang* will not be possible. Then the master cannot give his grace to you. Not that he will prevent himself from giving; you are not available. He cannot do anything, you are not open.

The sun may be waiting near the window but if it is closed, what can the sun do? The rays will reflect back. They will come, knock on the door, and go back. Remember, it is not a condition that you open the door and the sun will rise, it is not a condition! The sun may not be there, it may be night. Just by opening your door you cannot create the sun. Your opening of the door is just your being available: if the sun is there it can enter.

So seekers will move, will have to move from one master to another. The only thing to remember is that they must remain open and they should not judge. If you come near a master and you don't feel any tuning with him, move, but don't judge, because your judgment will be wrong. You have never been in contact. Unless you love you don't know, so don't judge. Simply say, "This master is not for me, I am not for this master. The thing has not happened." You simply move.

If you start judging then you are closing yourself for other masters also. You may have to pass through many, many situations, but remember this: don't judge. Whenever you feel that something is wrong with the master, move on. That means you cannot trust. Something has gone wrong, you cannot trust. But don't say the master is wrong, because you don't know! You simply move on, that's enough. You seek somewhere else.

If you start judging, condemning, concluding, then you will be closed. And the eyes which judge will never be able to trust. Once you have become a victim of judgment you will never be able to trust because you will find something or other which will help you not to trust, which will give you a closing.

So don't trust, don't judge, move on. Someday, if you go on moving, the thing is bound to happen. Someday, somewhere, in some moment – because there are moments; you cannot do anything about them. When you are vulnerable and when the master is flowing you meet. In a certain point of time and space, the meeting happens. Then *satsang* becomes possible.

Satsang means to be in close proximity with a master, with a man who has known, because then he can flow. He is already flowing. Sufis say that that's enough; just to be in close proximity to a master is enough. Just to sit near him, just to walk by his side, just to sit outside his room, just to watch in the night sitting outside his wall, just to go on remembering, that is enough.

But it takes years, many years of waiting. And he will not treat you well, remember – he will create every type of hindrance. He will give you many chances to judge. He will spread rumors about himself so you can think that he is wrong and you can escape. He will help you in every way to escape. Unless you pass all these necessary hurdles, and they are necessary because a cheap trust is of no use – it needs a seasoned trust which has waited long and has become a strong rock – only then can the deepest layers be penetrated.

Patanjali doesn't say that you will have to believe. Belief is intellectual. You believe in Hinduism, it is not your trust. It is just that accidentally you were born in a Hindu family. And so you have heard; from the very childhood you have been impregnated. You have been impressed with theories, concepts, philosophies, systems. They have become part of your blood. They have just fallen into your unconscious, you believe in them. But that belief is of no use because it has not transformed you, it is a dead thing, borrowed.

Trust is never a dead thing. You cannot borrow trust from your family; it is a personal phenomenon. *You* will have to come to it. Hinduism is traditional, Mohammedanism is traditional.

That's why the *sangham,* the first group around Mohammed, were the real Mohammedans because it was a trust for them; they had come personally to the master. They had lived with the master in close proximity, they had *satsang.* They believed in Mohammed, and Mohammed is not a man to be easily trusted – difficult. If you had been to Mohammed you would have had to resist him, it was impossible to believe in such a man. He had nine wives. He had a sword in his hand and on his sword was written, "Peace is the motto"; the word *islam* means peace. How can you believe this man?

You can believe in a Mahavira when he says, "Nonviolence"; he *is* nonviolent. Obviously, you can believe in Mahavira. How can you believe in Mohammed with a sword? And he says, "Love is the message and peace is the motto." You cannot believe. This man is creating hurdles.

He was a Sufi; he was a master. He would create every difficulty. So if your mind still functioned, you doubted, you were skeptical, you could escape. But if you remained, waited, if you had patience – and infinite patience would have been needed – someday you would come to know Mohammed, you would become a Mohammedan. Just by knowing him you would become a Mohammedan.

The first group of disciples was a totally different thing. The first group of disciples of Buddha was a totally different thing. Now Buddhists are dead, Mohammedans are dead. They are traditionally Mohammedans.

Truth cannot be transferred like property. Your parents cannot give you truth. They can give you property because the property belongs to the world. Truth doesn't belong to the world, they cannot give it to you; they cannot have it as a treasure. They cannot have it in the bank so that it can be transferred to you. You will have to seek on your own. You will have to suffer and you will have to become a disciple and you will have to pass through rigorous discipline. It will be a personal happening. Truth is always personal: it *happens* to a person. Trust is different, belief is different. Belief is given by others, trust is earned by you.

Patanjali doesn't require any belief. But without trust nothing can be done, without trust nothing is possible. But you cannot force it. Understand, you cannot force your trust; it is not in your hands to force it. If you force, it will be false, and no trust is better than a false trust, because you are wasting yourself. It is better to move somewhere else where the real can happen.

Don't judge, go on moving: someday, somewhere, your master is waiting. And the master cannot be shown to you – "Go here and this will be your master." You will have to seek, you will have to suffer, because through suffering and seeking you will be able to see him. Your eyes will become clear. The tears will disappear, your eyes will be unclouded and you will realize that this is the master.

It is reported that one of the Sufis named Junnaid went to an old fakir and said to him, "I have heard that you know. Show me the path."

The old man said, "You have *heard* that I know. *You* don't know. Look at me and feel."

The man said, "I cannot feel anything. Just do one thing, just show me the path where I can find my master."

So the old man said, "Go first to Mecca. Do the pilgrimage and search for such and such a man. He will be sitting under a tree. His eyes will be such, they will be throwing light, and you will feel a certain perfume like musk around him. Go and seek."

And Junnaid traveled and traveled for twenty years. Wherever he heard there was a master, he would go. But neither was the tree there, nor the perfume, the musk, nor those eyes the old man has described. The personality was not there. And he had a ready-made formula, so he would judge immediately, "This is not my master," and he would move on. After twenty years he reached under a tree – the master was there. The musk was floating in the air just like a haze around the man. The eyes were fiery, a red light was flowing. This was the man! He fell at his feet and said, "Master, I have been searching for you for twenty years."

The master said, "I have also been waiting for you for twenty years. Look again."

He looked, and saw that this was the same man who twenty years before had told him the way to find the master. Junnaid started weeping. He said, "What? You played a joke on me? Twenty years wasted! Why couldn't you have said that you are my master?"

The old man said, "That would not have helped. That would not have been of any use because you did not have eyes to see. These twenty years helped *you* to see me. I am the same man, but twenty years ago you told me 'I don't feel anything.' I am the same, but now you have become capable to feel. You have changed. These twenty years rubbed you hard – all the dust has fallen, your mind is clear. This fragrance of musk was also there that time but you were not capable of smelling it. Your nose was closed, your eyes were not functioning, and your heart was not really beating so contact was not possible."

You don't know, and nobody can say where the trust will happen. I don't say trust the master. I simply say find the person where trust happens – that person is your master. And you cannot do anything about it. You will have to wander. The thing is certain to happen, but the seeking is necessary because seeking prepares you. Not that the seeking leads you to the master: seeking prepares you so that you can see. He may be just near you...

The fifth question:

Osho,
Last night you spoke of satsang and the importance of

the disciple's proximity to the guru. Does this mean
physical proximity? Is the disciple who lives at a
great physical distance from the guru at a loss?

Yes and no. Yes, a physical closeness is necessary in the beginning because as you are, you cannot understand anything else right
now. You can understand the body, you can understand the language
of the physical. You exist at the physical, so yes, a physical closeness
is necessary in the beginning.

And I also say no, because as you grow, as you start learning a
different language which is of the non-physical, then physical closeness is not necessary. Then you can go anywhere. Then space doesn't
make any difference, you remain in contact. Not only space, but time
also doesn't make any difference. A master may be dead, you remain
in contact. He may have dropped his physical body, you remain in
contact. If a trust happens, then both time and space are transcended.

Trust is the miracle. You can be in closeness with Mohammed or
Jesus or Buddha right now if trust is there. But it is difficult because
you don't know how. You cannot trust a living person, how can you
trust a dead one? But if trust happens, then you are close to Buddha
right now. And for persons who have faith, Buddha is alive. No
master ever dies for those who can trust. He goes on helping, he is
always there. But for you, even if Buddha is there physically standing
behind you or in front of you, just sitting by your side, you are not
close to him. There may be vast space between you. Love, trust,
faith destroy both space and time.

In the beginning, because you cannot understand any other language, you can understand only the language of the physical, physical closeness is necessary – but only in the beginning. A moment will
come when the master himself will send you away. He will force you
to go away because that too becomes necessary or you may start
clinging to the physical language.

All of his life, Gurdjieff nearly always sent his disciples away. He
would create such a miserable situation for them that they would
have to leave. It would be impossible to live with him. After a certain
point he would help them to go away. He would really force them to
go away, because one should not become too much dependent on
the physical. The other, the higher language, must develop. You
must start feeling close to him wherever you are, because the body

has to be transcended. Not only your body, but the master's body also has to be transcended.

But in the beginning physical closeness is a great help. Once the seeds are sown, once they have taken root, then you are strong enough. Then you can go away and still you can feel. If just by going away the contact is lost, then the contact is not of much importance. Trust will grow more the further away you go. Trust will grow more, because wherever you are on the earth you will start feeling the master's presence continuously. The trust will grow. He will be helping you now through hidden hands, invisible hands. He will be working on you through your dreams and you will feel that constantly, like a shadow, he is following you.

But that is a very developed language. Don't try it from the very beginning because then you can deceive yourself. So I will say, move step by step. Wherever trust happens, then close your eyes and follow blindly. Really, the moment trust happens you have closed your eyes. Then what is the use of thinking, arguing? Trust has happened and trust will not listen to anything now. Then follow, and remain close unless the master himself sends you away. And when he sends you away then don't cling. Then follow his instruction and go away, because he knows better. And he knows what is helpful.

Sometimes just being near the master may make it difficult for you to grow, just as under a big tree a new seed will have many difficulties to grow. Under a big tree a new tree will become crippled. Even trees take care to throw their seed far away so that the seeds can sprout. The trees use many tricks to send the seed away. Otherwise they will die if they fall down just under the big tree; there is so much shadow, no sun reaches there, no sunrays reach.

So a master knows better. If he feels that you should go away, then don't resist. Then simply follow and go away. This going away will be a coming nearer to him. If you can follow, if you can silently follow without any resistance, then this going away will be a coming nearer. You will attain a new closeness.

The sixth question:

Osho,
When you ask us to understand something clearly, whom do you address to understand? Mind has to cease.

> Therefore, it is no use trying to make the mind
> understand anything. Who should understand then?

Yes, mind has to cease, but it has not ceased yet. Mind has to be worked on. An understanding has to be created in the mind: through that understanding this mind will die. That understanding is just like poison: you take the poison – you are the taker and the poison kills you. The mind understands, but the understanding is poison for the mind. That's why the mind resists so much. It tries and tries not to understand, it creates doubt, it fights. In every way it protects itself because understanding is poison for the mind. It is elixir for you, but for the mind it is poison.

So when I say understand clearly, I mean your mind, not you, because *you* need not have any understanding, you are already understanding. You are the very wisdom, the *pragnya*. You need no help from me or from anybody else.

Your mind has to be changed. And if understanding happens to the mind, mind will die, and with the mind the understanding will disappear. Then you will be in your purity; your being will reveal a mirror-like purity – no content, contentless. But that inner being needs no understanding; it is already the very core of understanding. It needs no understanding, just the clouds of the mind have to be persuaded.

Really, understanding is just a persuasion for the mind to leave. Remember, I don't say fight, I say persuasion. If you fight, the mind will never leave because through fight you show your fear. If you fight you show that the mind is something you are afraid of. Just persuade. All these teachings, all meditations are a deep persuasion for the mind to come to a point where it can commit suicide, where it simply drops, where mind itself becomes such an absurdity that you cannot carry it anymore – you simply drop it. It is better to say mind drops itself.

So when I say clear understanding, I am addressing your mind. And there is no other way. Only your mind can be approached because *you* are unavailable. You are so hidden deep inside, and just the mind is at the door. The mind has to be persuaded to leave the door and to leave the door open so you will become available.

I am addressing mind – your mind, not you. If mind drops there is no need to address. I can sit in silence and you will understand; there is no need to address. The mind needs words, the mind needs thoughts, the mind needs something mental which can persuade it. When Buddha or Patanjali or Krishna talk to you, they are addressing your mind.

A moment comes when mind simply becomes aware of the whole absurdity. It is just like this: I see that you are pulling the strings of your shoelaces, trying to pull yourself up by them, and I tell you, "What nonsense you are doing! This is impossible. You cannot pull yourself up just by your own shoelaces. It is simply impossible, it cannot happen." So I persuade you to think more about the whole thing: "This is absurd. What are you doing?" And then you feel miserable because it is not happening. So I go on telling you, insisting, hammering, and one day you may become aware, "Yes, this is absurd. What am I doing?"

The whole effort of the mind is just like pulling yourself up by your own shoelaces. Whatsoever you are doing is absurd. It can never lead you anywhere other than to hell, than to misery. It has always led you to misery, but you are still not aware. All this communication from me is just to make your mind alert that the whole effort is absurd. Once you come to feel that the whole effort is absurd, the effort disappears. It is not that you will have to leave your shoelaces and you will have to make some effort and it is going to be arduous: you will simply see the fact and you will stop and you will laugh. If you drop your shoelaces and simply stand and laugh, you have become enlightened. This is going to be the case.

Through understanding the mind drops. Suddenly you become aware that no one else was responsible for your misery, you were creating it; continuously, moment to moment, you were the creator. And you were creating the misery and then you were asking how to go beyond it, how to not be miserable, how to achieve bliss, how to achieve samadhi. And even as you are asking, you are creating. Even this asking, "How to achieve samadhi?" is creating misery because then you say, "I have been making so much effort and samadhi has not been attained yet. I am doing everything that can be done and the samadhi has not been attained yet. When will I become enlightened?"

Now you create a new misery when you make enlightenment also an object of desire, which is absurd. No desire will come to a fulfillment. When you realize this, desires drop – you are enlightened. Desireless, you are enlightened. With desires you go moving in a circle of misery.

The last question:

> Osho,
> You said that Yoga is a science, a methodology for inner
> awakening. But effort to be, to go nearer to no-mind,
> implies motivation and hope. Even to undergo the
> process of inner transformation implies motivation.
> Then how can one move on the path of Yoga without
> hope and motivation? Does not waiting even imply
> motivation?

Yes, you cannot move on the path of Yoga with motivation, with desire, with hope. Really, there is *no* movement on the path of Yoga. When you come to understand that all desire is absurd, all desire is misery, then there is nothing to do, because every doing will be a new desire. There is nothing to do! You simply cannot do anything because whatsoever you do will lead you into a new misery. Then you don't do. Desires have dropped, mind has ceased, and this is Yoga. You have entered. This is not a movement, this is a stillness. Problems arise because of language. When I say that you have entered, it appears that you have moved. All movement ceases when desire ceases. You are in Yoga: *Now the discipline of Yoga.*

With motivation, in the name of Yoga you will again create other miseries. Every day people come to me and they say: "I have been practicing Yoga for thirty years, nothing has happened." But who told you that something is going to happen? You must be waiting for something to happen, that's why nothing has happened. Yoga says, don't wait for the future.

You meditate, but you meditate with the motive that through meditation you will reach somewhere, some goal. You are missing the point. Meditate and enjoy it! There is no goal, there is no future, no further; there is nothing ahead. Meditate, enjoy it without any motivation, and suddenly the goal is there. Suddenly the clouds disappear because they were created by your desire. Your motivation is the smoke which creates the clouds, and they have disappeared. So play with the meditation; enjoy it. Don't make it a means. It is the end. This is the whole point to be understood.

Don't create new desires. Understand the very nature of desire – that it is misery. Just try to understand the nature of desire and you will come to know that it is misery. Then what is to be done? Nothing is to be done! Becoming alert that desire is misery, desire drops: *Now the discipline of Yoga.* You have entered the path.

And it depends on your intensity. If your realization that desire is misery is so deep, so total, you have not only entered Yoga, you have become a *siddha*. You have reached the goal. It will depend on your intensity. If the intensity is total then you have reached the goal. If your intensity is not so total you have entered the path.

Enough for today.

five modifications of mind

The modifications of the mind are five.
They can be either a source of misery or of non-misery.

They are right knowledge, wrong knowledge,
imagination, sleep and memory.

Mind can be either the source of bondage or the source of freedom. Mind becomes the gate for this world, the entry; it can also become the exit. Mind leads you to hell, mind can also lead you to heaven. So it all depends on how the mind is used. Right use of mind becomes meditation; wrong use of the mind becomes madness.

Mind is there, with everyone. The possibility of darkness and light are both implied in it. Mind itself is neither the enemy nor the friend. You can make it a friend, you can make it an enemy; it depends on you, on the you who is hidden behind the mind. If you can make the mind your instrument, your slave, the mind becomes the passage through which you can reach the ultimate. If you become the slave and the mind is allowed to be the master, then this mind which has become the master will lead you to ultimate anguish and darkness.

All the techniques, all the methods, all the paths of Yoga, are really deeply concerned only with one problem: how to use the mind. Rightly used, mind comes to a point where it becomes no-mind. Wrongly used, mind comes to a point where it is just a chaos, many voices antagonistic to each other, contradictory, confusing, insane.

The madman in the madhouse and Buddha under his *bodhi* tree have both used the mind, both have passed through the mind. Buddha has come to a point where mind disappears. Rightly used, it goes on disappearing; a moment comes when it is not. The madman has also used the mind. Wrongly used, mind becomes divided; wrongly used, mind becomes many; wrongly used, it becomes a multitude. And finally the mad mind is there, you are absolutely absent.

Buddha's mind has disappeared and Buddha is present in his totality. A madman's mind has become total and he himself has disappeared completely. These are the two different poles. You and your mind: if they exist together then you will be in misery. Either you will have to disappear or the mind will have to disappear. If the mind disappears then you achieve truth; if you disappear you achieve insanity. And this is the struggle: who is going to disappear? Are you going to disappear, or the mind? This is the conflict, the root of all struggle.

These sutras of Patanjali will lead you step by step towards this understanding of the mind: what it is, what types of modes it takes, what types of modifications come into it, how you can use it and go beyond it. And remember, you have nothing else right now except the mind, you have to use it. Wrongly used you will go on falling into more and more misery.

You *are* in misery. That is because for many lives you have used your mind wrongly and the mind has become the master; you are just a slave, a shadow following the mind. You cannot say to the mind, "Stop!" You cannot order your own mind; your mind goes on ordering you and you have to follow it. Your being has become the shadow and the slave, an instrument.

Mind is nothing but an instrument, just like your hands or your feet. You order your feet and your legs to move and they move. When you say stop, they stop. You are the master. If I want to move my hand, I move it. If I don't want it to move, I don't move it. The hand cannot say to me, "Now I want to be moved." The hand cannot say to me, "Now I will move. Whatsoever you do, I am not going to listen to you." And if my hand starts moving in spite of me, then it will be a chaos in the body. The same has happened in the mind.

You don't want to think and the mind goes on thinking. You want to sleep – you are lying down on your bed, changing sides; you want to go to sleep and the mind continues. The mind says, "No, I am going to think about something"; you go on saying, "Stop!" and it never listens to you. And you cannot do anything. Mind is also an instrument but you have given it too much power. It has become dictatorial, and it will struggle hard if you try to put it in its right place.

Buddha also uses the mind, but his mind is just like your legs. People come to me and they ask, "What happens to the mind of an enlightened one? Does it simply disappear? He cannot use it?"

It disappears as a master, it remains as a slave. It remains as a passive instrument. If a Buddha wants to use it, he can use it. When Buddha speaks to you he will have to use it, because there is no possibility of speech without the mind. The mind has to be used. If you go to Buddha and he recognizes you – that you have also been before – he has to use the mind: without mind there can be no recognition, without mind there is no memory. But *he* uses the mind, remember – this is the distinction – and *you* are being used by the mind. Whenever he wants to use it, he uses it. Whenever he doesn't want to use it, he doesn't use it. It is a passive instrument that has no hold upon him.

So Buddha remains like a mirror. If you come before the mirror, the mirror reflects you. When you move the reflection is gone, the mirror is vacant. You are not like a mirror. You see somebody: the man has gone but the thinking continues, the reflection continues. You go on thinking about him, and even if you want to stop, the mind won't listen.

Mastery of the mind is Yoga. And when Patanjali says, "Cessation of the mind," he means cessation as a master. Mind ceases as a master. Then it is not active, then it is a passive instrument. You order, it works; you don't order, it remains still. It is just waiting, it cannot assert by itself. The assertion is lost, the violence is lost. It will not try to control you: now just the reverse is the case.

How to become masters? And how to put mind in its right place where you can use it, where if you don't want to use it you can put it aside and it remains silent? So the whole mechanism of the mind will have to be understood. Now we should enter the sutra.

The first sutra:

> *The modifications of the mind are five.*
> *They can be either a source of misery or of non-misery.*

The first thing to be understood: mind is not something different from the body, remember. Mind is part of the body. It *is* body, but deeply subtle; a state of body, but very delicate, very refined. You cannot catch it, but through the body you can influence it. If you take a drug, if you take LSD or marijuana or alcohol or something else, the mind is suddenly affected. The alcohol goes into the body, not into the mind, but the mind is affected. Mind is the subtlest part of the body.

The reverse is also true: influence the mind and the body is affected. That happens in hypnosis. A person who cannot walk, who says that he has a paralysis, can walk under hypnosis. You don't have paralysis, but if under hypnosis it is said, "Now your body is paralyzed, you cannot walk," you cannot walk. A paralyzed man can walk under hypnosis. What is happening? Hypnosis goes into the mind, the suggestion goes into the mind then the body follows.

So the first thing to be understood: mind and body are not two. This is one of the deepest discoveries of Patanjali. Now modern science recognizes it, it is very recent in the West. Now they say body-and-mind, but to talk in this dichotomy is not right. Now they say it is "psychosoma," it is mind-body. These two terms are just two functions of one phenomenon. One pole is mind, the other pole is body, so you can work from either and change the other.

The body has five organs of activity, five *indriyas,* five instruments of activity. The mind has five modifications, five modes of function. Mind and body are one. Body is divided into five functions, mind is also divided into five functions. We will go into each function in detail.

The second thing about this sutra is:

> *They can be either a source of misery or of non-misery.*

These five modifications of the mind, this totality of the mind, can lead you into deep anguish, in *dukkha,* in misery. Or if you rightly use this mind, its functioning, it can lead you into non-misery.

That word *non-misery* is very significant. Patanjali doesn't say that it will lead you into *ananda,* into bliss, no; at the most it can lead you into non-misery. The mind can lead you into misery if you wrongly use it, if you become a slave to it. If you become the master the mind can lead you into non-misery – not into bliss, because bliss is your nature; the mind cannot lead you to it. But if you are in non-misery then the inner bliss starts flowing.

The bliss is always there inside, it is your intrinsic nature. It is nothing to be achieved and earned, it is nothing to be reached some-where. You are born with it, you have it already, it is already the case. That's why Patanjali doesn't say that the mind can lead you into misery and can lead you into bliss, no. He is very scientific, very accurate. He will not use even a single word which can give you any untrue information. He simply says either misery or non-misery.

Buddha also says many times, whenever seekers will come to him – and seekers are after bliss, so they will ask Buddha, "How can we attain to the bliss, the ultimate bliss?" He will say, "I don't know. I can show you the path which leads to non-misery, just the absence of misery. I don't say anything about the positive, bliss, just the neg-ative. I can show you how to move into the world of non-misery."

That's all that methods can do. Once you are in the state of non-misery the inner bliss starts flowing. But that doesn't come from the mind, that comes from your inner being. So mind has nothing to do with it, mind cannot create it. If mind is in misery then mind becomes a hindrance; if mind is in non-misery then mind becomes an opening, but it is not creative, it is not doing anything.

You open the windows and the rays of the sun enter: by opening the windows you are not creating the sun, the sun was already there. If it were not there then just by opening the windows, rays wouldn't enter. Your window can become a hindrance: the sunrays may be outside and the window is closed. The window can hinder or it can give way. It can become a passage but it cannot be creative. It cannot create the rays, the rays are there.

Your mind, if it is in misery, becomes closed. Remember, one of the characteristics of misery is closedness. Whenever you are in misery you become closed. Observe – whenever you feel some anguish you are closed to the world. Even to your dearest friend you are closed. Even to your wife, your children, your beloved, you are closed when you are in misery, because misery gives you a shrinking inside. You shrink. From everywhere you have closed your doors.

That's why in misery people start thinking of suicide. Suicide means total closure, no possibility of any communication, no possibility of any door. Even a closed door is dangerous, someone can open it. So destroy the door, destroy all possibilities. Suicide means, "Now I am going to destroy all possibility of any opening. Now I am closing myself totally."

Whenever you are in misery you start thinking of suicide. Whenever you are happy you cannot think of suicide, you cannot imagine, you cannot even think that people would commit suicide. "Why? Life is such joy, life is such a deep music, why do people destroy life?" It appears impossible.

Why, when you are happy, does it look impossible? Because you are open, life is flowing in you. When you are happy you have a bigger soul, it expands; when you are unhappy you have a smaller soul, it shrinks.

When someone is unhappy touch him, take his hand into your hand, and you will feel the hand is dead; nothing is flowing through it, no love, no warmth. It is just cold, as if it belonged to a corpse. When someone is happy touch his hand: there is communication, energy is flowing. His hand is not just a dead end; his hand has become a bridge. Through his hand something comes to you, communicates, relates, a warmth flows. He reaches to you; he makes every effort to flow into you and he allows you also to flow within him.

When two persons are happy they become one. That's why oneness happens in love and lovers start feeling that they are not two. They are two, but they start feeling they are not two because in love they are so happy that a melting happens. They melt into each other, they flow into each other. Boundaries dissolve, definitions are blurred and they don't know who is who. In that moment they become one.

When you are happy you can flow into others and you can allow others to flow into you: this is what celebration means. When you allow everybody to flow in and you flow into everybody, you are celebrating life. And celebration is the greatest prayerfulness, the highest peak of meditation.

In misery you start thinking of committing suicide; in misery you start thinking of destruction. In misery you are at just the opposite pole of celebration. You blame, you cannot celebrate, you have a grudge against everything. Everything is wrong and you are negative and you cannot flow. You cannot relate and you cannot allow anybody to flow into you. You have become an island, closed completely. This is a living death. Life is only when you are open and flowing, when you are unafraid, fearless, open, vulnerable, celebrating.

Patanjali says mind can do two things. It can create misery. You can use it in such a way that you can become miserable, and you have used it this way, you are past masters of it. There is no need to talk about it, you know it already. You know the art of creating misery. You may not be aware, but that is what you are doing continuously. Whatsoever you touch becomes a source of misery; I say, whatsoever!

I see poor men, they are miserable, obviously, they are poor, the basic needs of life are not fulfilled. But then I see rich men who are also miserable, and these rich men think that wealth leads nowhere. That is not right. Wealth can lead to celebration, but you don't have the mind to celebrate. If you are poor you are miserable, if you become rich you are more miserable. The moment you touch the riches you have destroyed them.

You have heard the Greek story of the king Midas? Whatsoever he would touch would turn into gold. You touch gold, immediately it becomes mud. It is turned into dust and then you think that there is nothing in this world, even riches are useless. They are not useless, but your mind cannot celebrate, your mind cannot participate in any non-misery. If you are invited into heaven you will not find a heaven there, you will create a hell. As you are, wherever you go you will take your hell with you.

There is one Arabic proverb: that hell and heaven are not geographical places, they are attitudes. And no one enters heaven or hell – everybody enters *with* heaven or hell. Wherever you go you have your hell projection or the heaven projection with you. You have a projector inside: immediately you project.

But Patanjali is careful: he says misery or non-misery – positive misery or negative misery – but not bliss. Mind cannot give you bliss; no one can give it. It is hidden in you. When mind is in a non-miserable state, that bliss starts flowing. It is not coming from the mind, it is coming from beyond. That's why he says they can be either a source of anguish or of non-anguish.

The second sutra:

The modifications of the mind are five....

They are right-knowledge, wrong-knowledge,
imagination, sleep and memory.

The first is *praman,* right-knowledge. The Sanskrit word *praman* is very deep and really cannot be translated. Right-knowledge is just a shadow, not the exact meaning, because there is no word which can translate *praman. Praman* comes from the root *prama.* Many things have to be understood about it.

Patanjali says that the mind has a capacity: if that capacity is directed rightly then whatsoever is known is true, it is self-evidently true. We are not aware about it because we have never used it. That faculty has remained unused. It is just as if you come into a dark room, you have a torch, but you are not using it so the room remains dark. You go on stumbling onto this table, onto that chair, and you have a torch but the torch has to be switched on. Once you put the torch on, immediately darkness disappears, and wherever the torch is focused at least you know that spot becomes evident, self-evidently clear.

Mind has a capacity of *praman,* of right-knowledge, of wisdom. Once you know it, how to put it on, then wherever you move that light, only right-knowledge is revealed. Without knowing it, whatsoever you know will be wrong.

Mind has the capacity of wrong-knowledge also. In Sanskrit that wrong-knowledge is called *viparyaya,* false, *mithya.* And you have that capacity also. You take alcohol, what happens? – the whole world becomes a *viparyaya,* the whole world becomes false. You start seeing things which are not there. What has happened? Alcohol cannot create things. Alcohol is doing something within your body and brain. The alcohol starts working the center Patanjali calls *viparyaya.* The mind has a center which can pervert anything. Once that center starts functioning everything is perverted.

I am reminded...

Once it happened that Mulla Nasruddin and his friend were

drinking in a pub. They came out, completely drunk. Nasruddin was an old, experienced drinker; the other was new, so the other was affected more. The other asked, "Now I cannot see, I cannot hear, I cannot even walk rightly. How will I reach my home? Tell me, Nasruddin. Please direct me. How should I reach my home?"

Nasruddin said, "First you go. After so many steps you will come to a point where there are two ways: one goes to the right, the other goes to the left. You go to the left, because that which goes to the right doesn't exist. I have been many times on that right path also, but now I am an experienced man. You will see two paths – choose the left one, don't choose the right. That right one doesn't exist. Many times I have gone on it and then you never reach, you never reach your home."

Nasruddin was teaching his son the first lesson of drinking. The son was asking, he was curious; he asked, "When is one to stop?"

Nasruddin said, "Look at that table. Four persons are sitting there. When you start seeing eight, stop!"

The boy said, "But father, there are only two persons sitting there!"

Mind has a faculty. That faculty functions when you are under the influence of any drug, any intoxicant. Patanjali calls that faculty *viparyaya*, wrong-knowledge, the center of perversion.

Exactly opposite to it there is a center which you don't know. Exactly opposite to it there is another center: if you meditate deeply, silently, that other center will start functioning. That center is called *praman*, right-knowledge. Through the functioning of that center, whatsoever is known is right. So it is not a question of what you know; from *where* you know is the question.

That's why all the religions have been against alcohol. It is not on any moralistic grounds, no. It is because alcohol influences the center of perversion. And every religion is for meditation because meditation means creating more and more stillness, becoming more and more silent.

Alcohol does quite the opposite. It makes you more and more agitated, excited, disturbed; a trembling enters within you. The drunkard cannot even walk rightly; his balance is lost. Balance is lost not only in the body, but in the mind also.

Meditation means gaining the inner balance. When you gain the inner balance and there is no trembling, the whole body-mind has become still – then the center of right-knowledge starts functioning. Through that center, whatsoever is known is true.

Where are you? You are not alcoholics, you are not meditators; you must be somewhere between the two. You are not in any center. You are between these two centers of wrong-knowledge and right-knowledge. That's why you are confused.

Sometimes you have glimpses. You lean a little towards the right-knowledge center, then certain glimpses come to you. You lean toward the center which is of perversion, then perversion enters in you. And everything is mixed, you are in chaos. That's why either you will have to become meditators or you will have to become alcoholics, because confusion is too much and these are the two ways.

Either you lose yourself into intoxication... Then you are at ease because at least you have gained a center – maybe of wrong-knowledge, but you are centered. The whole world may say you are wrong, you don't think so; you think the whole world is wrong. At least in those moments of unconsciousness you are centered, centered in the wrong center, but you are happy because even centering in the wrong center gives a certain happiness. You enjoy it, hence, the great appeal of alcohol.

Governments have been fighting alcohol for centuries. Laws have been made, prohibition and everything, but nothing helps. Unless humanity becomes meditative, nothing can help. People will go on finding new ways and new means to get intoxicated. They cannot be prevented, and the more you try to prevent them, the more prohibition laws, the more appeal.

America did it and had to fall back. They tried their best, but when alcohol was prohibited more alcohol was used. They tried, they failed. India has been trying since Independence. It has failed, and many states have started again. It seems useless.

Unless man changes inwardly, you cannot force man by any prohibition; it is impossible, because then man will go mad. This is his way of remaining sane. For a few hours he becomes drugged, "stoned," then he is okay. Then there is no misery, then there is no anguish. The misery will come, the anguish will come, but at least it is postponed. Tomorrow morning the misery will be there, the anguish will be there, and he will have to face it. But by the evening he can hope again; he will drink and be at ease.

These are the two alternatives. If you are not meditative then sooner or later you will have to find some drug. And there are subtle drugs. Alcohol is not very subtle, it is very gross. There are subtle drugs. Sex may become a drug for you, and through sex you may be just losing your consciousness. You can use anything as a drug. Only meditation can help. Why? – because meditation gives you centering on the center which Patanjali calls *praman*.

Why does every religion put so much emphasis on meditation? Meditation must be doing some inner miracle. This is the miracle: that meditation helps you to put on the light of right-knowledge. Then wherever you move, then wherever your focus moves, whatsoever is known is true.

Buddha has been asked thousands and thousands of questions. One day somebody asked him, "We come with new questions. We have not even put the question before you and you start answering. You never think about it. How does it happen?"

So Buddha said, "It is not a question of thinking. You put the question and I simply look at it, and whatsoever is true is revealed. It is not a question of thinking and brooding about it. The answer is not coming as a logical syllogism. It is just a focusing of the right center."

Buddha is like a torch. Wherever the torch moves, it reveals. Whatsoever the question, that is not the point. Buddha has the light, and whenever that light will come on any question the answer will be revealed. The answer will come out of that light. It is a simple phenomenon, a revelation.

When somebody asks you, you have to think about it. But how can you think if you don't know? If you know there is no need to think. If you don't know what will you do? You will search in the memory, you will find many clues. You will just do a patchwork. You don't really know, otherwise the response would have been immediate.

I have heard...

A woman teacher in a primary school asked the children, "Have you any questions?"

One small boy stood and said, "I have one question and I have been waiting...whenever you ask I will ask it: what is the weight of the whole earth?"

She became disturbed because she had never thought about

it, never read about it. What is the weight of the whole earth? So she played a trick teachers know. They have to play tricks. She said, "Yes, the question is significant. Now tomorrow, everybody has to find the answer." She needed time. "Tomorrow I will ask the question, and for whoever brings the right answer there will be a present for him."

All the children searched and searched, but they couldn't find the answer. And the teacher ran to the library. The whole night she searched, and only just by the morning could she find out the weight of the earth. She was very happy. She came back to school and the children were there. They were exhausted. They said they couldn't find the answer. "We asked Mom and we asked Dad and we asked everybody. Nobody knows. This question seems to be so difficult."

The teacher laughed and she said, "This is not difficult. I know the answer, but I was just trying to see whether you could find it out or not. This is the weight of the earth..."

That small child who had raised the question, he stood again and he asked, "With people or without?" Now the same situation...

You cannot put Buddha in such a situation. It is not a question of finding somewhere; it is not really a question of answering you. Your question is just an excuse. When you put a question to Buddha, he simply moves his light towards that question and whatsoever is revealed is revealed. He answers you, that is a deep response of his right-center, *praman*.

Patanjali says there are five modifications of the mind. Right-knowledge: if this center of right-knowledge starts functioning in you, you will become a sage, a saint. You will become religious. Before that you cannot become religious.

That's why Jesus and Mohammed look mad – because they don't argue; they don't put their case logically, they simply assert. You ask Jesus, "Are you really the only son of God?" He says, "Yes." And if you ask him, "Prove it," he will laugh. He will say, "There is no need to prove it. I know. This is the case, this is self-evident." To us it looks illogical. This man seems to be neurotic, claiming something without any proof.

If *praman*, this center of *prama*, this center of right-knowledge starts functioning, you will be the same: you can assert but you cannot prove. How can you prove? If you are in love how can you prove that you are in love? You can simply assert. You have a pain in your leg: how can you prove that you have pain? You simply assert, "I have pain." You know somewhere inside; that knowing is enough.

Ramakrishna was asked, "Is there a God?"
He said "Yes."
He was asked, "Then prove it."
He said, "There is no need – I know. For me there is no need. For you there is a need, so you search. Nobody could prove it for me, I cannot prove it for you. I had to seek, I had to find. And I have found God is!"

This is the functioning of the right center. So Ramakrishna or Jesus look absurd: they are claiming certain things without giving any proof. They are not claiming, they are not claiming anything. Certain things are revealed to them because they have a new center functioning which you don't have – and because you don't have it you need proof.

Remember, proving proves that you don't have an inner feeling of anything, everything has to be proved; even love has to be proved. And people go on...

I know many couples: the husband goes on proving that he loves and he has not convinced the wife, and the wife goes on proving that she loves and she has not convinced the husband. They remain unconvinced and that remains the conflict. They keep feeling that the other has not yet proved it. Lovers go on searching. They create situations in which you have to prove that you love. And by and by both get bored – this futile effort to prove and nothing can be proved.

How can you prove love? You can give presents, but nothing is proved. You can kiss and hug and you can sing, you can dance, but nothing is proved. You may be just pretending.

This first modification of the mind is right-knowledge. Meditation leads to this modification. And when you can know rightly and there is no need to prove, only then can mind be dropped, not before it. When there is no need to prove, mind is not needed because mind is a logical instrument. You need it every moment. You have to think, find what is wrong and what is right. Every moment there are choices and alternatives; you have to choose.

Only when *praman* functions, when right-knowledge functions, can you drop the mind, because now choosing has no meaning. You move choicelessly; whatsoever is right is revealed to you.

The definition of a sage is one who never chooses. He never chooses good against bad. He simply moves towards the direction which is that of good. It is just like sunflowers: when the sun is in the east the flower turns to the east, it never chooses; when the sun moves to the west the flower turns to the west. It simply moves with the sun. It has not chosen to move, it has not decided; it has not taken a decision, "Now I should move because the sun has moved to the west."

A sage is just like a sunflower – he simply moves wherever good is. So whatsoever he does is good. The Upanishads say, "Don't judge sages. Your ordinary measurements won't do." You have to choose good against bad. He has nothing to choose, he simply moves; whatsoever he does is good. And you cannot change him because it is not a question of alternatives. If you say, "This is bad," he will say, "Okay, it may be bad, but this is how I move, this is how my being flows."

Those who knew – and people in the days of the Upanishads knew – had decided that, "We will not judge a sage." Once a person has come to be centered in himself, when a person has achieved meditation, has become silent and the mind has been dropped, he is beyond our morality, beyond tradition. He is beyond our limitations. If we can follow we can follow him, if we cannot follow we are help-less. But nothing can be done and we should not judge.

If right-knowledge functions, if your mind has taken the modifi-cation of right-knowledge, you will become religious. Look, it is totally different. Patanjali doesn't say if you go to the mosque, to the *gurudwara,* to the temple, if you do some ritual, you pray... No, that's not religion. You have to make your right-knowledge center function, so whether you go to the temple or not is immaterial; it doesn't matter. If your right-knowledge center functions, whatsoever you do is prayerfulness and wherever you go is a temple.

Kabir has said, "Wherever I go I find you, my God. Wherever I move, I move into you, I stumble upon you. And whatsoever I do, even walking, eating, it is prayer." Kabir says, "This spontaneity is my *samadhi.* Just to be spontaneous is my meditation."

Second is wrong-knowledge: if your center of wrong-knowledge is functioning, then whatsoever you do you will do wrongly, and whatsoever you choose you will choose wrongly. Whatsoever you decide will be wrong because you are not deciding, the wrong center is functioning.

There are people who feel very unfortunate because whatsoever they do goes wrong. And they try not to do wrong again, but that's not going to help because their center has to be changed. Their mind functions in a wrong way. They may think that they are doing good but they will do bad. With all their good wishes they cannot help it; they are helpless.

Mulla Nasruddin used to visit a saint. He visited for many, many days. And the saint was a silent one, he would not say anything. Then Mulla Nasruddin had to ask; he said, "I have been coming again and again, waiting that you will say something. And you have not said anything. And unless you speak I cannot understand. So just give me a message for my life, a direction so I can move in that direction."

So that Sufi sage said, "*Neki kar kuyen may dal*": Do good, and throw it in the well. It is one of the oldest Sufi sayings: "Do good, and throw it in the well." It means do good and forget it immediately; don't carry the thought, "I have done good."

So next day Mulla Nasruddin helped one old woman to cross the road, and then he pushed her into the well.

Neki kar kuyen may dal: Do good, and throw it in the well.

If your wrong center is functioning, whatsoever you do – you can read the Koran, you can read the Gita, and you will find such meanings that Krishna would be shocked, Mohammed would be shocked to see that you could find such meanings.

Mahatma Gandhi wrote his autobiography with the intention of helping people. Then many letters came to him because he describes his sex life. He was honest, one of the most honest men, so he wrote everything, whatsoever had happened in his past: how he was too indulgent the day his father was dying; he couldn't sit by his father's side even that day, he had to go with his wife to bed.

The doctors had told him, "This is the last night. Your father cannot survive till the morning. He will be dead by the morning." But just about twelve or one in the night Gandhi started feeling desire, sexual desire. The father was feeling sleepy so Gandhi slipped away, went to his wife and indulged in sex. And the wife was pregnant, it was the ninth month. The father was dying, he died in the night, and the child also died at the moment of birth. So his whole life Gandhi had a deep repentance that he couldn't be with his dying father because sex was so obsessive.

So he wrote everything, he was honest – and just to help others. But many letters started coming to him, and those letters were such that he was shocked. Many people wrote to him, "Your autobiography is such that we have become more sexual than before reading it. Just reading through your autobiography we have become more sexual and indulgent. It is erotic."

If the wrong center is functioning then nothing can be done. Whatsoever you do, read, behave, it will be wrong. You will move to the wrong. You have a center which is forcing you to move towards the wrong. You can go to Buddha, but you will see something wrong in him immediately. You cannot meet Buddha – immediately you will see something wrong. You have a focusing for the wrong, a deep urge to find wrong anywhere, everywhere.

Patanjali calls this modification of the mind *viparyaya*. *Viparyaya* means perversion. You pervert everything; you interpret everything in such a way that it becomes a perversion.

Omar Khayyam writes, "I have heard that God is compassionate." This is beautiful. Mohammedans go on repeating, "God is *rahman*, compassion; *rahim*, compassion." They go on repeating, continuously. So Omar Khayyam says, "If he is really compassionate, if he is compassion, then there is no need to be afraid. I can go on committing sin. If he is compassion then what is the fear? I can commit whatsoever sin I want and he is compassion – so whenever I stand before him I will say, '*Rahim, rahman*: Oh God of compassion, I have sinned... But you are compassion; if you are really compassion then have compassion on me.'" So he goes on drinking, he goes on committing whatsoever he thinks is sin. He has interpreted in a very perverted way.

All over the world people have done that. In India we say, "If you go to the Ganges, if you bathe in the Ganges, your sins will dissolve." It was a beautiful concept in itself. It shows many things. It shows that sin is not something very deep, it is just like dust on you. So don't get too obsessed by it, don't feel guilty; it is just dust and inside you remain pure. Even bathing in the Ganges can help. This is just to show you not to become so obsessed with sin the way Christianity has become. Guilt has become so burdensome, so even just taking a bath in the Ganges will help. Don't be so afraid. But how have we interpreted it? We say, "Then it is okay – go on committing sin." And after a while, when you feel that now you have committed many sins, so give a chance to the Ganges to purify them and then come back and commit again. This is the center of perversion.

Third is imagination: mind has the faculty to imagine. It is good, it is beautiful. All that is beautiful has come through imagination. Paintings, art, dance, music, everything that is beautiful has come through the imagination. But everything that is ugly has also come through the imagination. Hitler, Mao, Mussolini, have all come through imagination.

Hitler imagined a world of supermen. And he believed in Friedrich Nietzsche who had said, "Destroy all those who are weak. Destroy all those who are not super; leave only supermen on the earth." So he destroyed. Just imagination, just utopian imagination – that just by destroying the weak, just by destroying the ugly, just by destroying the physically crippled you will have a beautiful world. But the very destruction is the ugliest thing possible in the world – the very destruction.

But he was working through imagination. He had an imagination, a utopian imagination; he was the most imaginative man! Hitler is one of the most imaginative men ever, and his imagination became so fantastic and so mad that for his imagined world he tried to destroy this world completely. His imagination had gone mad.

Imagination can give you poetry and painting and art, and imagination can also give you madness. It depends on how you use it. All the great scientific discoveries have been through imagination – people who could imagine, who could imagine the impossible. Now we can fly into the air, now we can go to the moon. These are deep imaginings.

Man has been imagining for centuries, millennia, how to fly, how to go to the moon. Every child is born with the desire to go to the moon, to catch the moon. But we reached it! Through imagination creativity comes, but through imagination destruction also comes.

Patanjali says imagination is the third mode of mind. You can use it in a wrong way and then it will destroy you. You can also use it in a right way. And then there are imaginative meditations: they start with imagination, but by and by imagination becomes subtler and subtler and subtler. And then imagination is ultimately dropped and you are face to face with the truth.

All Christian and Mohammedan meditations are basically through imagination. First you have to imagine something, then you go on imagining it and then through imagination you create an atmosphere around you. Try it; try what is possible through imagination. Even the impossible is possible.

If you think you are beautiful, if you imagine you are beautiful, a certain beauty will start happening to your body. So whenever a man says to a woman, "You are beautiful," the woman changes immediately. She may not have been beautiful before this moment. She may not have been beautiful, just homely, ordinary, but this man has given imagination to her.

So every woman who is loved becomes more beautiful, every man who is loved becomes more beautiful. A person who is not loved may be beautiful, but becomes ugly because he cannot imagine, she cannot imagine. And if imagination is not there, you shrink.

Coué, one of the great psychologists of the West, helped millions of people to be cured of many, many diseases just through imagination. His formula was very simple. He would say, "Just start feeling that you are okay. Just go on repeating inside the mind, 'I am getting better and better. Every day I am getting better.' In the night, while you fall asleep, go on thinking you are healthy, and you are getting healthier every moment, and by the morning you will be the healthiest person in the world. Go on imagining."

And he helped millions of people. Even incurable diseases were cured. It looked like a miracle. It is nothing but a basic law: your mind follows imagination.

Now psychologists say that if you say to children, "You are duffers, dull," they become dull. You force them to be dull. You give their imagination the suggestion that they are dull.

Many experiments have been done. Say to a child, "You are dull. You cannot do anything; you cannot solve this mathematical problem," and give him the problem and tell him, "Now try" – he will not be able to solve it. You have closed the door. Say to the child, "You are intelligent and I have not seen any boy as intelligent as you; for your stage, for your age you are over-intelligent. You show many potentialities, you can solve any problem. Now try this" – and he will be able to solve it. You have given imagination to him.

Now these things are scientifically proven, scientifically discovered, that whatsoever imagination catches becomes a seed. Whole generations have been changed, whole ages; whole countries have been changed just through imagination.

Go to the Punjab...

I was traveling once from Delhi to Manali. My driver was a Sikh, a sardar. The way, the road, was dangerous, and the car was very big. And many times the driver became afraid. Many times he would say, "Now I cannot go ahead. We will have to go back."

We tried in every way to persuade him. At one point he became so afraid he stopped the car, got out of the car and said, "No! Now I cannot move from here. It is dangerous." He said. "It may not be dangerous for you, you may be ready to die. But I am not, I want to go back."

By chance one of my friends who is also a sardar and a big police official was also coming. He was following me to attend the camp in Manali. His car arrived and I told him, "Do something! The man has got out of the car."

That police official came and he said, "You are a sardar, a Sikh, and a coward? Get into the car!"

The man immediately got into the car and started it. So I asked him, "What is the matter?"

He said, "Now he has touched my ego. He says, 'You are a sardar?' – Sardar means leader of men – 'a Sikh and a coward?!' He has touched my imagination. He has touched my pride. Now we can go. Dead or alive, we will reach Manali!"

And this has not only happened with one man. In the Punjab it has happened with millions. Look at the Hindus of the Punjab and at the Sikhs of the Punjab. Their blood is the same, they belong to the same race, just five hundred years ago all were Hindus. And then a different type of race, a military race, was born. Just by growing a beard, just by changing your face, you cannot become brave. But you can with imagination. Nanak gave them the imagination that, "You are a different type of race. You are unconquerable." And once they believed, once that imagination started to work, within five hundred years a new race, totally different from Punjabi Hindus, came into being in the Punjab. Nothing is different, but in India no one is braver than they. These two world wars have proved that on the whole of the earth, Sikhs have no comparison. They can fight fearlessly.

What has happened? Just their imagination has created a milieu around them. They feel that just by being Sikhs they are different. Imagination works! It can make a brave man out of you, it can make you a coward.

I have heard...

Mulla Nasruddin was sitting in a pub, drinking. He was not a brave man, one of the most cowardly, but alcohol gave him courage. And then a man, a giant of a man, entered the pub. He was ferocious looking, dangerous, looked like a murderer. At any other time, in his senses, Mulla Nasruddin would have been afraid, but now he was drunk so he was not afraid at all.

That ferocious looking man went near to Mulla, and seeing that he was not afraid at all he stomped on his feet. Mulla got angry, furious, and he said, "What are you doing? Are you doing it on purpose or is it just a sort of joke?" But by this time, by stomping on his feet, Mulla was brought back from his alcohol. He was brought back, he came to his senses. But he had said, "What are you doing? Is it on purpose or is it just a sort of joke?"

The man said, "On purpose."

Mulla Nasruddin said, "Then thank you. On purpose it is okay, because I don't like those types of jokes"

Patanjali says imagination is the third faculty. You go on imagining... If you wrongly imagine you can create delusions around you, illusions, dreams, and you can be lost in them. LSD and other drugs help and work on this center. So whatsoever potentiality you have inside, your LSD trip will help you develop it. So nothing is certain. If you have happy imaginations, the drug trip will be a happy trip, a high. If you have miserable imaginations, nightmarish imaginations, the trip is going to be bad.

That's why many people make contradictory reports. Huxley says it can become a key to the door of heaven, and Rheiner says it is ultimate hell. It depends on you; LSD cannot do anything. It simply jumps on your center of imagination and starts functioning there chemically. If you have an imagination of the nightmarish type then you will develop that, and you will pass through hell. And if you are addicted to beautiful dreams you may reach heaven.

This imagination can function either as a hell or as heaven. You can use it to go completely insane. What has happened to madmen in the madhouses? They have used their imagination, and they have used it in such a way that they are engulfed by it. A madman may be sitting alone and he is talking loudly to someone. He not only talks, he answers also. He questions, he answers, he speaks for the other who is absent also. You may think that he is mad, but he is talking to a real person. In his imagination the person is real, and he cannot judge what is imaginary and what is real.

Children cannot judge. So many times children may lose their toy in a dream, and then they will weep in the morning, "Where is my toy?" They cannot judge that a dream is a dream and reality is reality. And they have not lost anything, they were just dreaming. The boundaries are blurred; they don't know where the dream ends and where reality starts.

A madman is also blurred. He doesn't know what is real, what is unreal. If imagination is used rightly then you will know that this is imagination, and you will remain alert that this is imagination. You can enjoy it, but this is not real.

So when people meditate, many things happen through their imagination. They start seeing lights, colors, visions, talking to God himself, or moving with Jesus or dancing with Krishna. These are imaginative things, and a meditator has to remember that these are functions of the imagination. You can enjoy it, nothing is wrong in them, they are fun, but don't think that they are real.

Remember that only the witnessing consciousness is real, nothing else is real. Whatsoever happens may be beautiful – enjoy, enjoy it. It is beautiful to dance with Krishna, nothing is wrong in it. Dance, enjoy, but remember continuously that this is imagination, a beautiful dream. Don't get lost in it. If you are lost in it then imagination has become dangerous. Many religious people are just in imagination and they move into imagination and waste their life.

The fourth faculty is sleep. Sleep means unconsciousness as far as your outward-moving consciousness is concerned. It has gone deep into itself. Activity has stopped, conscious activity has stopped.

Mind is not functioning. Sleep is a non-functioning of the mind. If you are dreaming then it is not sleep. You are just in the middle between waking and sleep. You have left waking and you have not entered sleep; you are just in the middle.

Sleep means a totally contentless state – no activity, no movement in the mind. Mind has been completely absorbed, relaxed. This sleep is beautiful, it is life-giving. You can use it. And this sleep, if you know how to use it, can become *samadhi*. Samadhi and sleep are not very different. There is only one difference: in *samadhi* you will be aware; everything else will be the same.

In sleep everything is the same, only you are not aware. You are in the same bliss into which Buddha entered, in which Ramakrishna lives, in which Jesus has made his home. In deep sleep you are in the same blissful state, but you are not aware. So in the morning you feel the night has been good, in the morning you feel refreshed, vital, rejuvenated. In the morning you feel that the night was just beautiful, but this is just an afterglow. You don't know what has happened, what really happened. You were not aware.

Sleep can be used in two ways. Just as a natural rest... You have even lost that. People are not really going into sleep – they go on dreaming continuously. Sometimes, for a very few seconds, they touch deep sleep, and they again start dreaming. The silence of sleep, the blissful music of sleep, has become unknown, you have destroyed it. Even natural sleep is destroyed. You are so agitated and excited that the mind cannot fall completely into oblivion.

But Patanjali says natural sleep is good for the body's health, and if you can become alert in sleep it can become *samadhi*, it can become a spiritual phenomenon. So there are techniques – we will discuss them later on – of how sleep can become an awakening. The Gita says that the yogi doesn't sleep even while he is asleep. He remains alert, something inside goes on being aware. The whole body falls into sleep, the mind falls into sleep, but the witnessing remains. Someone is watching – a watcher on the tower goes on. Then sleep becomes *samadhi*; it becomes the ultimate ecstasy.

And the fifth modification of the mind is memory. That too can be used or misused. If memory is misused it creates confusion. Really, you may remember something, but you cannot be certain whether it happened that way or not. Your memory is not reliable. You may add many things to it; imagination may enter into it. You may delete many things from it, you may do many things to it. And when you say, "This is my memory," it is a very refined and changed thing. It is not real.

Everybody says, "My childhood was just paradise" – and look at children. These children will also say later on that their childhood was paradise, and they are suffering. And every child hankers to grow up soon, to become an adult. Every child thinks that adults are enjoying, they are enjoying all that is worth enjoying. They are powerful, they can do everything; he is helpless. Children think they are suffering. But these children will grow as you have grown, and then later on they will say that childhood was beautiful, just a paradise.

Your memory is not reliable. You are imagining. You are just creating your past. You are not true to it. And you drop many things from it – you drop all that was ugly, all that was sad, all that was painful; all that was beautiful you continue. You remember all that was a support to your ego, and all that was not a support you drop, you forget.

So everybody has a great storehouse of dropped memories. And whatsoever you say is not true because you cannot remember truly. All your centers are confused and they enter into each other and disturb.

Right-memory... Buddha has used the words *right-memory* for meditation. Patanjali says, if memory is right, that means one has to be totally honest with oneself. Then, only then, can memory be right. Whatsoever has happened, bad or good, don't change it. Know it as it is. It is very hard, it is arduous. You choose and change. Knowing one's past as it is will change your whole life. If you rightly know your past as it is, you will not like to repeat it in the future. Right now everybody is thinking of how to repeat it in a modified form, but if you know your past exactly as it was, you will not like to repeat it.

Right-memory will give you the impetus of how to be free from all lives. And if memory is right then you can even go into past lives. If you are honest then you can go into past lives. And then you have only one desire: to transcend all this nonsense. But you think the past was beautiful, and you think the future is going to be beautiful, only this present is wrong. But the past was present a few days before, and the future will become present a few days after. And each time each present is wrong and all past is beautiful and all future is beautiful. This is wrong memory. Look directly at the past, don't change it; look at the past as it was. But we are very dishonest.

Every man hates his father, but if you ask anybody he will say, "I love my father. I honor my father as no one else." Every woman hates her mother, but ask and every woman will say, "My mother is just divine." This is wrong-memory.

Gibran has a story. He says one night a mother and daughter were awakened suddenly by a noise. They both were sleepwalkers, and at the time the sudden noise happened in the neighborhood, they were both walking in the garden, asleep. They were sleepwalkers.

It must have been a shock, because in sleep the old woman, the mother, was saying to the daughter, "Because of you, you bitch – because of you my youth is lost. You destroyed me. And now anybody who comes to the house looks at you. Nobody looks at me." A deep jealousy that comes to every mother when the daughter becomes young and beautiful: it happens to every mother, but it is inside.

And the daughter was saying, "You old rotten... Because of you I cannot enjoy life. You are the hindrance. Everywhere you are the hindrance, the obstacle. I cannot love, I cannot enjoy."

And suddenly, because of the noise, they were both awakened. And the old woman said, "My child, what are you doing here? You may catch cold. Come inside."

And the daughter said, "But what are you doing here? You were not feeling well and this is a cold night. Come, mother. Come to bed."

The first thing that was happening was coming from the unconscious. Now they are again pretending. They have become awake. Now the unconscious has gone back and the conscious mind has come in. Now they are hypocrites. Your conscious mind is hypocrisy.

To be truly honest with one's own memories one will have to really pass through arduous effort. And you have to be true, whatsoever it is. You have to be nakedly true. You have to know what you really think about your father, about your mother, about your brother, about your sister – really. And don't mix, don't change, don't polish what you have in the past; let it be as it is. If this happens, then, Patanjali says, this will be a freedom. You will drop it. The whole thing is nonsense and you will not want to project it again into the future.

Then you will not be a hypocrite. You will be real, true, sincere.

You will become authentic. And when you become authentic you become like a rock: nothing can change you, nothing can create confusion.

You become like a sword: you can always cut whatsoever is wrong, you can divide whatsoever is right from the wrong. And then a clarity of mind is achieved. That clarity can lead you towards meditation. That clarity can become the basic ground to grow – to grow beyond.

Enough for today.

madness or meditation

The first question:

Osho,
You said that there are only two alternatives for man,
either madness or meditation. But millions of people on
the earth have not reached to either of the two. Do you
think they will?

They *have* reached. They have not reached to meditation, but
they have reached to madness. And the difference between
the mad who are inside the madhouses and the mad who are
outside the madhouses is only of degrees. There is no qualitative difference; the difference is only of quantity. You may be less mad,
they may be more mad, but man as he is, is mad.

Why do I say man as he is, is mad? Madness means many things.
One: you are not centered. If you are not centered you will be insane,
with many voices in you. Not centered, you are many, you are a multitude. And no one is a master in the house, and every servant of the
house claims to be the master. There is confusion, conflict and a continuous struggle. You are in a continuous civil war. If this civil war

were not going on then you would be in meditation. But it continues day and night, for twenty-four hours. Write down whatsoever goes on in your mind for a few minutes, and be honest. Write down exactly whatsoever goes on and you yourself will feel that this is mad.

I have a particular technique I use with many people. I say to them, sit in a closed room and then start saying loudly whatsoever comes into the mind. Talk aloud so that you can listen. After fifteen minutes of this talking, you will feel that you are listening to a madman. Absurd, inconsistent, unrelated fragments float in the mind, *your* mind! So you may be ninety-nine percent mad and someone else has crossed the boundary, he has gone beyond one hundred percent. Those who have gone beyond one hundred percent are put in the madhouses. We cannot put you in the madhouse because there are not enough madhouses. And there cannot be, or the whole earth would have to be a madhouse.

Khalil Gibran writes a small anecdote:

He says, one of his friends became mad so he was put in a madhouse. Then just out of love, compassion, Gibran went to see him, to visit him. He was sitting under a tree in the garden of the madhouse, surrounded by a very big wall. Khalil Gibran went there, sat by the side with his friend on the bench and asked him, "Do you ever think about why you are here?"

The madman laughed and he said, "I am here because I wanted to leave that big madhouse outside. And I am at peace here. In this madhouse – you call it a madhouse – no one is mad."

Mad people cannot think that they are mad; that is one of the basic characteristics of madness. If you are mad you cannot think that you are mad. If you can think you are mad there is a possibility that you may not be. If you can think and conceive that you are mad you are still a little sane. The madness has not occurred in its totality. So this is the paradox: those who are really sane know that they are mad, and those who are completely mad cannot think that they are mad.

You never think that you are mad: that is part of madness. You are not centered; you cannot be sane. Your sanity is just superficial, arranged. Just on the surface you appear to be sane. That's why you have to continuously deceive the world around you. You have to hide much, you have to prevent much. You don't allow everything to come out. You are suppressive: you may be thinking something but you will say something else. You are pretending, and because of this pretension you can have the minimum superficial sanity around you; inside you are boiling.

Sometimes there are eruptions. In anger you erupt and the madness that you have been hiding comes out. It breaks all your adjustments. So psychologists say anger is a temporary madness. You will again regain balance, you will again hide your reality, you will again polish your surface – you will again become sane. And you will say that, "It was wrong. I did it in spite of myself. I never meant it, so forgive me." But you meant it! That was more real! This asking for forgiveness is just a pretension. Again you are maintaining your surface, your mask.

A sane man has no mask. His face is original: whatsoever he is, he is. A madman has to continuously change his faces. Every moment he has to use a different mask for a different situation, for different relationships. Just watch yourself changing your faces: when you come to your wife you have one face, when you go to your beloved, your mistress, you have a totally different face. When you talk to your servant you have a different mask and when you talk to your master, a totally different face. It may be that your servant is standing on your right and your boss is standing on your left – then you have two faces simultaneously. On the left you have one face, on the right you have a different face. Because to the servant you cannot show the same face; you need not – you are the boss there, so one side of the face will be "the boss." You cannot show that "boss face" to your boss, you are a servant there; your other side will show a servile attitude.

This is constantly going on. You are not watching, that's why you are not aware. If you watch you will become aware that you are mad. You don't have any face; the original face has been lost. To regain the original face is what meditation means.

So Zen masters say, "Go and find your original face, the face you had before you were born, the face you will have when you have died." Between birth and death you have false faces, you continuously go on deceiving. Not only others, you also deceive yourself; when you stand before a mirror you deceive yourself, you never see your real face in the mirror. You don't have enough courage to face yourself. That face in the mirror is also false. You create it, you enjoy it; it is a painted mask.

We are not only deceiving others, we are also deceiving ourselves. Really, we cannot deceive others if we have not already deceived ourselves. So we have to believe in our own lies, only then can we make others believe. If you don't believe in your lies nobody else is going to be deceived.

This whole nuisance that you call your life leads nowhere. It is a mad affair. You work too much, you overwork; you walk and run. You struggle your whole life and you reach nowhere. You don't know from where you are coming, you don't know where you are moving to, where you are going. If you meet a man on the road and you ask him, "Where are you coming from, sir?" and he says, "I don't know," and you ask him, "Where are you going," and he says, "I don't know," and still he says, "Don't prevent me, I am in a hurry," what will you think about him? You will think he is mad.

If you don't know where you are coming from and where you are going, then what is the hurry? But this is the situation of everybody, and everybody is on the road. Life is a road – you are always in the middle – and you don't know where you have come from, you don't know where you are going. You have no knowledge of the source, no knowledge of the goal, but you are in a great hurry, making every effort to reach nowhere.

What type of sanity is this? And out of this whole struggle not even glimpses of happiness come to you, not even glimpses. You simply hope someday, somewhere, tomorrow, the day after tomorrow – or after death, in some afterlife – that happiness is waiting for you. This is just a trick to postpone, so that you don't feel too miserable right now.

You don't even have glimpses of bliss. What type of sanity is this? You are in continuous misery, and moreover, misery that is not created by anybody else. You create your suffering. What type of sanity is this? You create your suffering continuously. I call it madness.

Sanity will be this: you will become aware that you are not centered. So the first thing to be done is to get centered – to have a center within yourself from where you can lead your life, from where you can discipline your life; to have a master within you from where you can direct, you can move. The first thing is to be crystallized, and then the second thing will be not to create suffering for yourself. Drop all that creates suffering, all those motives, desires, hopes which create suffering.

But you are not aware. You simply go on doing it, you don't see that you create it. Whatsoever you do, you are sowing some seeds. Then trees will follow, and whatsoever you have sown you will reap. And whenever you reap anything there is suffering, but you never see that these seeds were sown by you. Whenever suffering happens to you, you think it is coming from somewhere else. You think it is some accident or that some evil forces are working against you. So you have invented the Devil.

The Devil is just a scapegoat. You are the Devil; you create your suffering. But whenever you suffer you simply throw it on the Devil: "The Devil is doing something." Then you are at ease. Then you never become aware of your own foolish pattern of life, stupid pattern of life.

Or you call it fate, or you say, "God is testing me." But you go on avoiding the basic fact that you are the sole cause of whatsoever happens to you. And nothing is accidental. Everything has a causal link – and you are the cause.

For example, you fall in love. Love gives you a feeling that bliss is somewhere nearby. You feel for the first time that you are welcomed by someone, at least one person welcomes you. You start flowering. Even one person welcoming you, waiting for you, loving you, caring for you, you start flowering. But only in the beginning, immediately your wrong patterns start working, and you immediately want to possess the beloved, the loved one.

And possession is killing. The moment you possess the lover you have killed. Then you suffer. Then you weep and cry and you think that the lover is wrong, fate is wrong, "Destiny is not in my favor." But you don't know that you have poisoned love through possession, through possessiveness.

But every lover is doing that, and every lover suffers. Love, which can give you the deepest blessings, becomes the deepest misery; therefore old cultures, particularly in India in the old days, completely destroyed the phenomenon of love. They had arranged marriages for children – no possibility of falling in love, because love leads to misery. This was such a known phenomenon that if you allow love, then love leads to misery, so it is better not to have the possibility. Let the children, small children, be married. Before they can fall in love let them be married. Then they will never know what love is and they will not be in misery.

But love never creates misery – it is you who poisons it. Love is always joy, love is always celebration. Love is the deepest ecstasy that nature allows you, but you destroy it. So just not to fall into misery, in India and in other old, ancient countries, the possibility of love was completely closed. So then you will not fall in misery, but then you have also missed the only ecstasy that nature allows. So a mediocre life will be there with no misery, no happiness, just dragging on somehow. This is what marriage has been in the past.

Now America is trying, the West is trying to revive love. But much misery is coming through that, and sooner or later Western countries will have to decide for child marriage again. A few psychologists have already proposed that child marriage has to be brought back because love is creating so much misery. But I say again that it is not love. Love cannot create misery. It is you, your pattern of madness which creates misery – and not only in love, everywhere. Everywhere you are bound to bring your mind.

For example, many people come to me, and they start meditating. In the beginning there are sudden flashes, but only in the beginning. Once they have known certain experiences, once they have known certain glimpses, everything stops. And they come to me weeping and crying and saying, "What is happening? Something was going to happen, something was happening, now everything has stopped. And we are trying our best, but nothing, nothing comes out of it."

I tell them, "It happened for the first time because you were not expecting. Now you are expecting so the whole situation has changed. When you had that feeling of weightlessness for the first time, a feeling of being filled by something unknown, a feeling of being carried from your dead life, a feeling of ecstatic moments, you were not expecting it. You had never known such moments. For the first time they were falling on you. You were unaware, unexpecting. That was the situation.

"Now you are remembering that situation, and every day you sit for meditation with expectation. Now you are cunning, clever, calculating. When for the first time you had the glimpse you were innocent, like a child. You were playing with meditation and there was no expectation. Then it happened. It will happen again but only when you have again become innocent. Now your mind is bringing misery.

And if you go on insisting that you must have the experience again and again, you will lose it forever. You must forget it completely. It may take years, unless you become again completely inattentive that somewhere in the past such a happening was there. Then the possibility will again be open to you."

This I call madness. You destroy everything, whatsoever comes in your hands, you immediately destroy it. And remember life gives you many gifts, unasked. You have never asked life. Life gives you many gifts, but you destroy every gift. And every gift can become greater and greater; it can grow because life never gives you anything dead. If love has been given to you it can grow. It can grow to unknown dimensions. But the very first moment you destroy. If meditation has happened to you just feel thankful to the divine and forget it. Just feel grateful and remember well that you don't have any capacity to have it; you are not in any way authorized to have it.

It has been a gift. It has been an overflowing of the divine. Forget it. Don't expect it, don't demand it. It will come some day again – deeper, higher, greater. It will go on expanding, but every day drop it from the mind.

There is no end to its possibilities. It will become infinite; the whole cosmos will become ecstatic for you. But your mind has to be dropped. Your mind is the madness. So when I say there are only two alternatives, madness and meditation, I mean mind and meditation. If you remain confined in the mind you will remain mad. Unless you transcend the mind you cannot transcend madness. At the most you can be a functioning member of the society, that's all. And you can be a functioning member of the society because the whole society is just like you. Everybody is mad, so madness is the rule.

Become aware – and don't think that others are mad; feel it deeply that you are mad and something has to be done. Immediately! It is an emergency! Don't postpone it because there may come a moment when you cannot do anything. You may go so mad that you cannot do anything.

Right now you can do something. You are still within limits. Something can be done, some efforts can be made; the pattern can be changed. But a moment can come when you cannot do anything, when you have become completely shattered and you have lost even the consciousness.

If you can feel that you are mad this is a very hopeful sign. It shows you can become alert towards your own reality. The door is there, you can become really sane. At least this much sanity is there – that you can understand.

The second question:

> Osho,
> Capacity of right-knowledge is one of the five faculties of the mind, but it is not a state of no-mind. Then how is it possible that whatsoever one sees through this center is true? Does this center of right-knowledge function after enlightenment, or can even a meditator, a sadhak, be with this center?

Yes, the center of right-knowledge, *praman,* is still within the mind. Ignorance is of the mind, knowledge is also of the mind. When you go beyond mind there is neither; there is neither ignorance nor knowledge. Knowledge is also a disease. It is a good disease, a golden one, but it is a disease. So really, it cannot be said that Buddha knows, it cannot be said that he doesn't know. He has gone beyond. Whether he knows or is ignorant, nothing can be asserted about it.

When there is no mind, how can you know or not know? Knowing is through mind, not knowing is also through mind. Through mind you can know wrongly, through mind you can know rightly. When there is no mind, knowledge and ignorance both cease. This will be difficult to understand, but it is easy if you follow: mind knows, so mind can be ignorant; when there is no mind how can you be ignorant and how can you be knowing? You are, but knowing and not knowing have both ceased.

Mind has two centers: one, of right-knowledge. If that center functions it starts functioning through concentration, meditation, contemplation, prayerfulness – then whatsoever you know is true. There is a wrong center: it functions if you are sleepy, live in a hypnotic-like state, intoxicated with something or other – sex, music, drugs or anything.

You can be addicted to food, then it becomes an intoxicant. You may be eating too much. You are mad, obsessed, with food. Then food becomes like alcohol. Anything that takes possession of your mind, anything without which you cannot live becomes intoxicating. So if you live through intoxicants then your center of wrong-knowledge functions and whatsoever you know is false, untrue. You live in a world of lies.

But both these centers belong to the mind. When mind drops and meditation has come to its totality... In Sanskrit we have two terms: one term is *dhyana* – *dhyana* means meditation; and the other term is *samadhi*. *Samadhi* means perfect meditation, where even meditation has become unnecessary, where even to do meditation is meaningless. You cannot do it, you have become it – then it is *samadhi*.

In this state of *samadhi* there is no mind; there is neither knowledge nor ignorance, there is only pure being. This pure being is a totally different dimension. It is not a dimension of knowing, it is a dimension of being.

Even if such a man as a Buddha or a Jesus wants to communicate to you, he will have to use mind. For communication he will have to use mind. And if you ask a certain question he will have to use his center of mind for right-knowledge. Mind is the instrument of communication, of thinking, of knowing.

But when you are not asking anything and Buddha is sitting under his *bo* tree, he is neither ignorant nor a knower. He is there. Really, there is no difference between the tree and the Buddha. There is a difference, but in a way there is no difference. He has become just as if a tree; he just exists. There is no movement, even of knowledge. The sun will rise but he will not *know* that the sun has risen. Not that he will remain ignorant – no, simply that is now not his movement. He has become so silent, so still, that nothing moves. He is just like the tree. The tree is totally ignorant. Or, you can say the tree is just below the mind; the mind has not started functioning. The tree will become man in some life, the tree will become mad like you in some life, and the tree will try for meditation in some life, and the tree will also one day become a buddha. The tree is below mind, and Buddha sitting under the tree is beyond mind. They are both mindless. One is still to attain the mind and one has attained and crossed over it.

So when mind is transcended, when no-mind is achieved, you are a pure being, *satchitananda*. There is no happening in you. Neither is there action nor is there knowing – but it is difficult for us...

Scriptures say that all duality is transcended. Knowledge is also part of duality – ignorance, knowledge. But so-called saints go on saying that Buddha had become "a knower." Then we are clinging to the duality. That's why Buddha never answered when many times, millions of times it had been asked of him, "What happens when a person becomes a buddha?" He remained silent. He said, "Become and know." Nothing can be said about what happens because what-soever can be said will be said in your language. And your language is basically dualistic so whatsoever can be said will be untrue.

If it is said that he knows it will be untrue, if it is said that he has become immortal it will be untrue, if it is said that now he has achieved bliss it will be untrue – because all duality disappears. Misery disappears, happiness disappears. Ignorance disappears, knowledge disappears. Darkness disappears, light disappears. Death disappears, life disappears. Nothing can be said. Or, only this much can be said – that whatsoever you can think will not be there, whatsoever you can conceive of will not be there. And the only way is, to become that. Only then do you know.

The third question:

Osho,
You said that if we see visions of Rama or that we are dancing with Krishna, to remember it is only imagination. But the other night you said that if we were receptive we could communicate with Christ, Buddha or Krishna right now. Is that communication also imagination when it happens, or are there meditative states in which Christ or Buddha are really there?

This is a little difficult to understand. The first thing: out of one hundred cases, ninety-nine cases will be of imagination. You imagine, which is why to a Christian Krishna never appears in visions; to a Hindu Mohammed never appears in visions. Leave Mohammed and Jesus; they are far away. But to a Jaina Rama never appears in his visions – cannot appear. To a Hindu Mahavira never appears. Why? – you don't have any imagination for Mahavira.

If you are born a Hindu you have been fed with the concept of Rama and Krishna. If you are born a Christian you have been fed – your computer, your mind, has been fed – with the image of Jesus. Whenever you start meditating that fed-in image comes up in the mind; it flashes in the mind.

Jesus appears to you, Jesus never appears to Jews. And he was a Jew. He was born a Jew, he died a Jew, but he never appears to Jews because they never believed in him. They thought he was just a vagabond, they crucified him as a criminal. Jesus never appears to Jews; he belonged to Jews, he had Jewish blood and bones.

I have heard...

In Nazi Germany soldiers of Hitler were killing Jews in a town. They had killed many. A few Jews escaped. It was a Sunday morning. They escaped; they went into a church because they thought that would be the best hiding place, the Christian church. The church was filled with Christians, it was a Sunday morning. So a few, a dozen Jews were hiding there.

But the soldiers got the news that some Jews had gone into the church and they were hiding there. So they went into the church; they told the priest, "Stop your service!" The leader of the soldiers went to the rostrum and said, "You cannot deceive us. There are a few Jews hiding here. So anyone who is a Jew should go out and stand in a line. If you follow our orders you can save yourself. If someone tries to deceive, he will be killed immediately."

So by and by, the Jews came out of the church and they stood in a line. Then suddenly the whole crowd in the church became aware that Jesus had disappeared, the statue of Jesus. He was also a Jew so he was standing outside in the line!

But Jesus never appears to Jews. He was not a Christian, he never belonged to any Christian church. If he comes back he will not recognize a Christian church, he will go to the synagogue; he will go to the Jewish community. He will go to see the rabbi; he cannot go to see a Catholic or Protestant priest. He doesn't know. But he never appears to Jews because he has never been a seed in their imagination. They refused him, so the seed is not there.

So whatsoever happens, ninety-nine possibilities are that it may be just fed-in knowledge, concepts, images: they flash before your mind. And when you start meditating you become sensitive. You become so sensitive that you can become a victim of your own imagination. And the imagination will look so real, and there is no way to judge whether it is real or unreal.

In one percent of cases it will not be imaginary, but how can you know? In that one percent of cases there will be no image, really. You will not feel Jesus standing before you crucified, you will not feel Krishna standing before you and dancing with you. You will feel the presence but there will be no image, remember this. You will feel a descendance of divine presence. You will be filled with something unknown, but without any form. There will be no dancing Krishna and there will be no crucified Jesus and there will be no Buddha sitting in *siddhasan,* no! There will simply be a presence, a vital presence that is flowing within you, in and out. You are overwhelmed, you are in the ocean of it.

Jesus will not be within you, you will be in Jesus; that will be the difference. Krishna will not be in your mind, an image; you will be in Krishna. But then Krishna will be formless. It will be an experience but not an image.

Then why call it Krishna? There will be no form. Why call it Jesus? These are simply symbols, linguistic symbols. You are acquainted with the word *Jesus* so when that presence fills you and you become part of it, a vibrating part of it, when you become a drop in that ocean, how can you express it? You know the most beautiful word for you may be *Jesus* or the most beautiful word may be *Buddha* or *Krishna* – these words are fed into the mind so you have to choose these certain words to indicate toward that presence.

But that presence is not an image, it is not a dream. It is not a vision at all. You can use Jesus, you can use Krishna, you can use Christ, or whatsoever name has appeal for you, whatsoever name has a love-appeal for you, that's up to you. That word and that name and that image will come from your mind, but the experience itself is imageless. It is not an imagination.

A Catholic priest was visiting a Zen master, Nan-in. Nan-in had never heard about Jesus, so this Catholic priest thought, "It will be good. I should go and read some parts from *The Sermon on the Mount,* and I will see how Nan-in reacts. And people say that he is enlightened."

So that Catholic priest went to Nan-in and he said, "Master, I am a Christian, and I have got a book and I love it. I would like to read something from it just to know how you respond, how you react." So he read a few lines from *The Sermon on the Mount,* The New

Testament. He translated it into Japanese because Nan-in could understand only Japanese.

When he started translating, the whole face of Nan-in changed completely. Tears started flowing from his eyes and he said, "These are the words of Buddha."

The Christian priest said, "No, no, these are the words of Jesus."

But Nan-in said, "Whatsoever name you give, I feel these are the words of the Buddha, because I know only Buddha and these words can come only through Buddha. And if you say they have come through Jesus, then Jesus was a buddha; that doesn't make any difference. Then I will tell my disciples that Jesus was a buddha."

This will be the feeling. If you feel the presence of the divine, then names are just immaterial. Names are bound to be different for everyone because names come from education, names come from culture, names come from the race you belong to. But that experience doesn't belong to any society, that experience doesn't belong to any culture, that experience doesn't belong to your mind, the computer – it belongs to you.

So remember, if you see visions, they are imagination. If you start feeling presences, formless, existential experiences – enveloped in them, merged in them, melting in them – then you are really in contact.

You can call that presence Jesus, you can call that presence Buddha, it depends on you; it makes no difference. Jesus is a buddha and Buddha is a christ. Those who have gone beyond the mind have also gone beyond personalities. They have also gone beyond forms. If Jesus and Buddha are standing together, there will be two bodies but one soul. There will be two bodies but not two presences, only one presence.

It is just as if you put two lamps in a room. There are two lamps, just their bodies, but the light has become one. You cannot demarcate that this light belongs to this lamp and that light belongs to that lamp. The lights have merged. Only the material part of the lamp has remained separate, but the non-material part has become one.

If Buddha and Jesus come close, if they stand together, you will see two lamps, separate, but their lights have already merged. They have become one. All those who have known truth have become one. Their names are different for their followers; for them, now there are no names.

The fourth question:

Osho,
Please explain whether awareness is also one of the
modifications of the mind.

No, awareness is not part of the mind. It flows through the mind, but it is not part of the mind. It is just like this bulb: the electricity flows through it, but the electricity is not part of the bulb. If you break the bulb you have not broken the electricity. The expression will be hindered, but the potentiality remains hidden. You put in another bulb and the electricity starts flowing.

Mind is just an instrument. Awareness is not part of it, but awareness flows through it. When mind is transcended, awareness remains in itself. That's why I say even Buddha will have to use the mind if he talks to you, if he relates to you, because then he will need flow, flow of his inner pool. He will have to use instruments, mediums, and then mind will function. But mind is just a vehicle.

You move in a vehicle, but you are not the vehicle. You go in a car or you fly in an aircraft, but you are not the vehicle. Mind is just the vehicle. And you are not using the mind to its total capacity. If you use it to its total capacity, it will become right-knowledge.

We are using our mind like someone using an airplane as a bus. You can cut the wings off the airplane and use it like a bus on the road. That will do, it will work like a bus – but you are foolish. That bus can fly! You are not using it to its right capacity.

You are using your mind for dreams, imaginations, madness. You have not used it rightly, you have cut the wings off. If you use it with the wings it can become right-knowledge, it can become wisdom. But that too is part of the mind, that too is the vehicle. The user remains behind; the user cannot be the used. *You* are using it, *you* are awareness. And all the effort for meditation is meant to know this awareness in its purity, without any medium, without any instrument. You can know it only when mind has stopped functioning. When mind has stopped functioning you will become aware that awareness is there, you are filled with it. Mind was just a vehicle, a passage. Now if you want you can use the mind, if you don't want you need not use it.

Body and mind are both vehicles. You are not the vehicle, you are the master hidden behind these vehicles. But you have forgotten completely. And you have become the cart, you have become the vehicle. This is what Gurdjieff calls identification. This is what in India yogis have called *tadatmya,* becoming one with something which you are not.

The fifth question:

Osho,
Please explain how it is possible that just by looking, by witnessing the recordings in the brain cells, the sources of thought-process can cease to be.

They never cease to be, but by witnessing identification is broken. Buddha lived in his body for forty years after his enlightenment, the body did not cease. Continuously, for forty years he was talking, explaining, making people understand what had happened to him and how the same can happen to them. He was using the mind, the mind had not ceased. And when he came back to his home town after twelve years he recognized his father, he recognized his wife, he recognized his son. The mind was there, the memory was there; otherwise recognition would have been impossible. The mind had not really ceased.

When we say the mind ceases, we mean your identification is broken. Now you know this is the mind and this is "I am." The bridge is broken. Now the mind is not the master. It has become just an instrument, it has fallen to its right place. So whenever you need it you can use it. It is just like this fan: if we want to use it we put it on, then the fan starts functioning. Right now we are not using the fan so it is non-functioning. But it is there, it has not ceased to be, any moment we can use it. It has not disappeared.

By witnessing identification disappears, not the mind. But by identification disappearing, you are a totally new being. For the first time you have come to know your real phenomenon, your real reality. For the first time you have come to know who you are. Now mind is just part of the mechanism around you.

It is just as if you are a pilot and flying an airplane: you use many instruments, your eyes are working on many instruments continuously aware of this and that, but you are not the instruments.

This mind, this body and many functions of the body-mind, are just around you – the mechanism. In this mechanism you can exist in two ways. One way of existence is forgetting yourself and feeling as if you are the mechanism. This is bondage, this is misery; this is the world, the *sansar.*

Another way of functioning is to become alert that you are separate, you are different. Then you go on using, but now it makes a lot of difference – now the mechanism is not you. And if something goes wrong in the mechanism you can try to put it right, but you will not be disturbed. Even if the whole mechanism disappears you will not be disturbed.

Buddha dying and you dying are two different phenomena. Buddha knows only the mechanism is dying. It has been used and now there is no need of it. A burden has been removed, he is becoming free. Now he will move without form. But you dying is totally different: you are suffering, you are crying because you feel *you* are dying, not the mechanism. It is *your* death; then it becomes an intense suffering.

Just by witnessing, mind doesn't cease and the brain cells will not cease. Rather, they will become more alive because there will be less conflict, more energy. They will become fresher, and you can use them more rightly, more accurately, but you will not be burdened by them and they will not force you to do something. They will not push and pull you here and there. You will be the master.

But how does it happen just by witnessing? – because the bondage has happened by *not* witnessing. The bondage has happened because you are not alert, so the bondage will disappear if you become alert. The bondage is only unawareness. Nothing else is needed but becoming more alert, whatsoever you do.

You are sitting here listening to me. You can listen with awareness, you can listen without awareness. Without awareness listening will also be there, but it will be a different thing, the quality will differ. Then your ears are listening and your mind is functioning somewhere else.

Then, somehow, a few words will penetrate you and they will be mixed, and your mind will interpret them in its own way. It will put its own ideas into them. Everything will be a muddle and a mess. You have listened but many things will be bypassed, you will not listen to many things, you will choose. Then the whole thing will be distorted.

If you are alert, the moment you become alert thinking ceases.

With alertness you cannot think. The whole energy becomes alert, there is no energy left to move into thinking. When you are alert even for a single moment, you simply listen. There is no barrier. Your own words are not there to get mixed in. You need not interpret. The impact is direct.

If you can listen with alertness, then what I am saying may be meaningful or may not be meaningful, but your listening with alertness will always be significant in meaning. That very alertness will make a peak of your consciousness. The past will dissolve, the future will disappear. You will be nowhere else, you will be just here and now.

In that moment of silence when thinking is not, you will be deep in contact with your own source. And that source is bliss, and that source is divine. So the only thing to be done is to do everything with alertness.

The last question:

Osho,
While talking on Lao Tzu you become a Taoist sage,
while talking on Tantra you become a tantrika, while
talking on bhakti you become an enlightened bhakta, and
while talking on Yoga you have become a perfect yogi.
Will you please explain how this phenomenon has
become possible?

If you are not, only then can it become possible. If you are, then it cannot become possible. If you are not, if the host has completely disappeared, then the guest becomes the host. So the guest may be Lao Tzu, the guest may be Patanjali. The host is not there, so the guest takes the place completely, he becomes the host. If you are not, then you can become Patanjali; there is no difficulty. You can become Krishna, you can become Christ. If *you* are there, then it is very difficult. And if *you* are there, whatsoever you say will be wrong.

That's why I say these are not commentaries. I am not commenting on Patanjali. I am simply absent, allowing Patanjali. So it is not a commentary.

"Commentary" means, "Patanjali is something separate, and I am something separate, and I am commenting on Patanjali" – it is bound to be distorted because how can you comment on Patanjali?

Whatsoever I say would be *my* saying, and whatsoever I say would be *my* interpretation. It cannot be of Patanjali himself. And that's not good. That is destructive. So I am not commenting at all. I am simply allowing, and this allowing is possible if you are not.

If you become a witness, the ego disappears. And when the ego disappears you become a vehicle, you become a passage, you become a flute. And the flute can be put on Patanjali's lips, and the flute can be put on Krishna's lips, and the flute can be put on Buddha's lips – the flute remains the same. But when it is on Buddha's lips, Buddha is flowing.

So this is not a commentary. This is difficult to understand because you cannot allow. You are so much inside you cannot allow anyone. And these are not persons. Patanjali is not a person: Patanjali is a presence. If you are absent, his presence can function.

If you ask Patanjali, he will say the same. If you ask Patanjali, he will not say that these sutras have been created by him. He will say, "These are very ancient – *sanatan*." He will say, "Millions and millions of seers have seen them. I am just a vehicle. I am absent and they are speaking." If you ask Krishna, he will say, "I am not speaking. This is the ancientmost message. It has been always so." And if you ask Jesus, he will say, "I am no more, I am not there."

Why this insistence? Anybody who becomes absent, who becomes a non-ego, starts functioning as a vehicle, as a passage for all that is true, a passage for all that is hidden in existence, that can flow. And you will be able to understand whatsoever I am saying only when even for a few moments you will be absent.

If you are too much there, your ego is there and then whatsoever I am saying cannot flow in you. It is not only an intellectual communication. It is something deeper.

If you are a non-ego even for a single moment, then the impact will be felt. Then something unknown has entered into you, and in that moment you will understand. And there is no other way to understand.

Enough for today.

CHAPTER 5

why can't you dance?

Right-knowledge has three sources: direct-cognition, inference and the words of the awakened ones,

Wrong-knowledge is a false conception not corresponding to the thing as it is.

An image conjured up by words without any substance behind it is vikalpa, imagination.

The modification of the mind which is based on the absence of any content in it, is sleep.

Memory is the calling up of past experiences.

The first sutra:

Right-knowledge has three sources: direct cognition, inference and the words of the awakened ones.

Pratyaksha, direct cognition, is the first source of right-knowledge. Direct cognition means a face-to-face encounter without any mediator, without any medium, without any agent. When you know something directly, the knower faces the known immediately. There is no one to relate, no bridge. Then it is right-knowledge. But then many problems arise.

Ordinarily, *pratyaksha,* direct cognition, has been translated, interpreted, commented on, in a very wrong way. The very word *pratyaksha* means before the eyes, in front of the eyes. But eyes themselves are a mediation, the knower is hidden behind. Eyes are the medium. You are hearing me but this is not direct, this is not immediate. You are hearing me through the senses, through the ears. You are seeing me through the eyes. Your eyes can wrongly report to you, your ears can wrongly report. No one should be believed; no mediator should be believed because you cannot rely on the mediator.

If your eyes are ill they will report differently, if your eyes are drugged they will report differently, if your eyes are filled with memory they will report differently. If you are in love then you see something that you can never see if you are not in love. An ordinary woman can become the most beautiful person in the world if you see through love. When your eyes are filled with love then they report something else. And the same person can appear ugly if your eyes are filled with hate. Eyes are not reliable.

You hear through the ears. Ears are just instruments, they can function wrongly; they can hear something which has not been said, they can miss something which was being said. Senses cannot be reliable, senses are just mechanical devices.

Then what is *pratyaksha,* what is direct cognition? Direct cognition can only be when there is no mediator, not even the senses. Patanjali says then it is right-knowledge. This is the first basic source of right-knowledge: when you know something and you need not depend on anybody else.

You transcend the senses only in deep meditation. Then direct cognition becomes possible. When Buddha comes to know his innermost being, that innermost being is *pratyaksha,* that is direct cognition. No senses are involved, nobody has reported it, there is no one like an agent. The knower and known are face to face, there is nothing in between. This is immediacy, and only immediacy can be true.

So the first right-knowledge can only be that of the inner self. You may know the whole world, but if you have not known the innermost core of your being all your knowledge is absurd, it is not really knowledge; it cannot be true because the first, basic, right-knowledge has not happened to you. Your whole edifice is false. You may know many things, but if you have not known yourself, all your knowledge is based on reports given by the senses. And how can you be certain that the senses are reporting rightly?

In the night you dream. While dreaming you start believing in the dream, that it is true. Your senses are reporting the dream: your eyes are seeing it, your ears are hearing it, you may be touching it. Your senses are reporting to you, that's why you fall under the illusion that it is real. You are here... It may be just a dream. How can you be certain that I am speaking to you, in reality? It is possible it may be just a dream, and you are dreaming me. Every dream is true while you dream.

Chuang Tzu once saw in a dream that he had become a butterfly. And in the morning he was sad. His disciples asked, "Why are you so sad?"

Chuang Tzu said, "I am in trouble. I have never been in such trouble before. This puzzle seems to be impossible, it cannot be solved. Last night I saw in a dream that I have become a butterfly."

The disciples laughed. They said, "What is there? This is not a riddle. A dream is just a dream."

Chuang Tzu said, "But listen, I am troubled. If Chuang Tzu can dream that he has become a butterfly, a butterfly may be dreaming now that she has become Chuang Tzu. So how to decide whether I am now facing reality or again a dream? And if Chuang Tzu can become a butterfly why can't a butterfly dream that she has become a Chuang Tzu?"

There is no impossibility, the reverse can occur. You cannot rely on the senses. In dreams the senses deceive you. If you take a drug, LSD or something, your senses will start deceiving you; you will start seeing things which are not there. They can deceive you to such an extent that you can start believing things so absolutely that you will be in danger.

One girl in New York jumped from the sixtieth floor because

under LSD she thought she could fly. Chuang Tzu was not wrong: the girl really flew out of the window. Of course, she died. But she will never be able to know that she had been deceived by her senses under the influence of the drug.

Even without drugs we have illusions. You are passing through a dark street and suddenly you get scared, you see a snake. You start running, and later on you come to know that there was no snake, just a rope was lying there. But when you felt that there was a snake, there *was* a snake. Your eyes were reporting that the snake was there and you behaved accordingly – you escaped from the place.

Senses cannot be believed. Then what is direct cognition? Direct cognition is something which is known without the senses. So the first right-knowledge can only be of the inner self, because only there will the senses not be needed. Everywhere else the senses will be needed. If you want to see me you will have to see through the eyes, but if you want to see yourself eyes are not needed. Even a blind man can see himself. If you want to see me light will be needed, but if you want to see yourself darkness is okay, light is not needed.

Even in the darkest cave you can know yourself. No medium, not light, eyes, nothing is needed. The inner experience is immediate, and that immediate experience is the basis of all right-knowledge.

Once you are rooted in that inner experience then many things will start happening to you. It will not be possible to understand them right now. One who is rooted in his center, in his inner being, one who has come upon it, to feel it as a direct experience, cannot be deceived by the senses. He is awakened, his eyes cannot deceive him, his ears cannot deceive him, nothing can deceive him. Deception has dropped.

You can be deceived because you are living in delusion. You cannot be deceived once you have come to be a right knower. You cannot be deceived! Then everything, by and by, takes the shape of right-knowledge. Once you know yourself, then whatsoever you know will automatically fall into being right because now *you* are right. This is the distinction to be remembered: if you are right then everything becomes right, if you are wrong then everything goes wrong. So it is not a question of doing something outside, it is a question of doing something inside.

You cannot deceive a buddha, it is impossible. How can you deceive a buddha? He is rooted in himself. You are transparent to him, you cannot deceive him. Before you know, he knows you. Even a glimmer of thought in you is clearly seen by him. He penetrates you to your very being.

Your penetration goes to the same extent in others as it goes into yourself. If you can penetrate into yourself, you can penetrate into everything to the same extent. The deeper you move within, the deeper you can move without. And you have not moved within even a single inch, so whatsoever you do outside is just like a dream.

Patanjali says the first source of right-knowledge is immediate, direct cognition, *pratyaksha*. He is not concerned with the *charvakas,* the old materialists, who said that only that which is before the eyes is true.

Because of this word *pratyaksha*, direct cognition, much misunderstanding has happened. The Indian school of materialists is Charvaka. The source of Indian materialism was Brihaspati, a very penetrating thinker, but a thinker; a very profound philosopher but a philosopher, not a realized soul. He says only *pratyaksha* is true, and by that he means whatsoever you know through the senses is true. And he says there is no way of knowing anything without the senses, so only sense-knowledge is real for *charvakas.*

Hence he denies there can be any God because no one has ever seen him. And only that which can be seen can be real, that which cannot be seen cannot be real. God exists not because you cannot see; the soul exists not because you cannot see it. And he says, "If there is a God, bring him before me so I can see him. If I see, then he is, because only seeing is truth." He also uses the word *pratyaksha*, direct cognition, but his meaning is totally different.

When Patanjali uses the word *pratyaksha* his meaning is on an altogether different level. He says immediate knowledge not derived from any instrument, not derived from any medium is true. And once this knowledge happens you have become true. Now nothing false can happen to you. When you are true, authentically rooted in truth, then illusions become impossible.

That's why it is said that buddhas never dream; one who is awakened never dreams – because even dreams cannot happen to him, he cannot be deceived. He sleeps, but not like you. He sleeps in a totally different way, the quality is different. Only his body sleeps, relaxes. His being remains alert, and that alertness won't allow any dreaming to happen.

You can dream only when alertness is lost. When you are not aware, when you are deeply hypnotized, then you start dreaming. Dreaming can happen only when you are completely unaware. The more unawareness, the more dreams there will be; the more awareness, the fewer dreams; fully aware, no dreams. Even dreaming becomes impossible for one who is rooted in himself, who has come to know the inner being immediately.

This is the first source of right-knowledge. The second source is inference. That is secondary, but that too is worth consideration because, as you are right now, you don't know whether there is a self within or not. You have no direct knowledge of your inner being. What to do? There are two possibilities. You can simply deny that there is an inner core of your being, there is no soul, as *charvakas* do, or in the West as Epicurus, Marx, Engels and others have done.

But Patanjali says that if you know, there is no need for inference, but if you don't know then too it will be helpful to infer. For example, Descartes, one of the greatest thinkers of the West, started his philosophical quest through doubt. He took the standpoint from the very beginning that he will not believe in anything which is not indubitable. That which could be doubted, he would doubt. And he would try to find a point which could not be doubted, and only on that point would he create the whole edifice of his thinking. It was a beautiful quest – honest, arduous, dangerous.

So he denied God, because you can doubt it. Many have doubted and no one has been able to answer their doubts. He went on denying. Whatsoever could be doubted, conceived to be dubitable, he denied. For years he was continuously in an inner turmoil. Then he fell upon the point which was indubitable: he couldn't deny *himself,* that was impossible. You cannot say, "I am not." If you say it, your very saying proves that you are. So this was the basic rock, "I cannot deny myself, I cannot say I am not. Who will say it? Even to doubt, I am needed."

This is inference. This is not direct cognition. This is through logic and argument, but it gives a shadow, it gives a glimpse, it gives you a possibility, an opening. And then Descartes had the rock, and on this rock a great temple can be built. One indubitable fact and you can reach to the absolute truth. If you start with a doubtful thing you will never reach anywhere. In the very base, doubt remains.

Patanjali says inference is the second source of right-knowledge.

Right-logic, right-doubting, right-argument can give you something which can help towards real knowledge. That he calls inference, *anuman*. You have not seen directly, but everything proves it; it must be so. There are situational proofs that it must be so.

For example, you look around the vast universe. You may not be able to conceive that there is a God, but you cannot deny; even through simple inference you cannot deny that the whole world is a system, a coherent whole, a design. That cannot be denied. The design is so apparent, even science cannot deny it. Rather, on the contrary, science goes on finding more and more designs, more and more laws.

If the world is just an accident then science is impossible. But the world doesn't seem to be an accident, it seems to be planned. And it is running according to certain laws and those laws are never broken.

Patanjali will say that design in the universe cannot be denied, and if once you feel there is design, the designer has entered. But that is an inference, you have not known him directly – but the design of the universe, the planning, the law, the order; and the order is so superb, it is so minute, so superb and so infinite, the order is there. Everything is humming with an order, a musical harmony of the whole universe. Someone seems to be hidden behind, but that's an inference. Patanjali says inference can also be a help towards right-knowledge, but it has to be right-inference. Logic is dangerous, it is double-edged. You can use logic wrongly, then too you will reach conclusions.

For example, I told you that the plan is there, the design is there; the world has an order, a beautiful order, perfect. Right-inference will be that there seems to be somebody's hand behind it. We may not be directly aware, we may not be in direct touch with that hand but a hand seems to be there, hidden. This is the right-inference.

But from the same premises you can also infer wrongly. There have been thinkers who have said as Diderot has said, "Because of order I cannot believe there is a God. In the world there seems to be perfect order. Because of this order, I cannot believe in God." What is his logic? He says if there is a person behind it, then there cannot be so much order. If a person is behind it then he must commit mistakes sometimes. Sometimes he must go whimsical, crazy, sometimes he will change. Laws cannot be so perfect if someone is behind them. Laws can be perfect if there is no one behind them and they are simply mechanical.

That too has an appeal. If everything goes perfectly, it looks mechanical because man is imperfect. It is said, to err is human. If some person is there then he must err sometimes; he will get bored with so much perfection. And sometimes he must like to change.

Water boils at one hundred degrees. It has been boiling at one hundred degrees for millennia, always and always. God must get bored. "So, if someone is behind," Diderot says, "just for a change, one day he will say, 'From now onwards the water will boil at ninety degrees.'" But it has never happened, so there seems to be no person.

Both arguments look perfect. But Patanjali says that right-inference is that which gives you possibilities of growth. It is not a question whether the logic is perfect or not. The question is your conclusion should become an opening. If there is no God it becomes a closing. Then you cannot grow. If you conclude there is some hidden hand, the world becomes a mystery. And then you are not here just by accident, your life becomes meaningful, you are part of a great scheme. Then something is possible, you can do something, you can rise in awareness.

A right-inference means one which can give you growth, that which can give you growth; a wrong-inference, howsoever perfect looking, is that which closes your growth. Inference can also be a source of right-knowledge. Even logic can be used to be a source of right-knowledge, but you have to be very aware of what you are doing. If you are just logical you may commit suicide through it. Logic can become a suicide, and for many it does become.

Just a few days ago a seeker from California was here. He had traveled a long way to come to meet me. He said, "Before I can meditate, or before you tell me to meditate – because I have heard that whosoever comes to you, you push them into meditation – so before you push me in, I have many questions." He had a list of at least a hundred questions. I think he had not left out any possible ones. He had questions about God, about the soul, about truth, about heaven and hell and everything – a sheet full of questions. He said, "Unless you solve these questions first, I am not going to meditate."

He is logical in a way because he says, "Unless my questions are answered how can I meditate? Unless I feel confident that you are right, you have answered my doubts, how can I go in a direction which you show and indicate? You may be wrong. So you can prove your rightness only if my doubts disappear."

Now his doubts are such that they cannot disappear. This is the dilemma: if he meditates they can disappear, but he says he will meditate only when these doubts are not there. What to do? He says, "First prove there is a God." No one has ever proved it, no one ever can. That doesn't mean that God is not there, but he cannot be proved. He is not a small thing which can be proved or disproved. It is such a vital thing that you have to live it to know it. No proof can help.

But logically he is right. He says, "Unless you prove, how can I start? If there is no soul, who is going to meditate? So first prove that there is a self, then I can meditate."

This man is committing suicide. No one will ever be able to answer him. He has created all the barriers, and through these barriers he will not be able to grow. But he is logical. What should I do with such a person? If I start answering his questions, a person who can create a hundred doubts can create millions, because doubting is a way, a style of mind. You can answer one question and through your answer he will create ten more questions because the mind remains the same.

He looks for doubts, and if I answer logically I am helping his logical mind to be fed, to be more strengthened. I am feeding it; that will not help. He has to be brought out of his logicalness.

So I asked him, "Have you ever been in love?"

He said, "But why? You are changing the subject."

I said, "I will come to your points, but suddenly it has become very meaningful to me to ask if you have ever loved."

He said, "Yes!" His face changed.

I asked, "But you loved before, or before falling in love, you doubted the whole phenomenon?"

Then he was disturbed. He was uncomfortable. He said, "No, I never thought about it. I had simply fallen in love, and only then I became aware."

So I said, "Do the opposite: first think about love, whether love is possible, whether love exists, whether love can exist. And first let it be proved. And make it a condition that unless it is proved you will not love anybody."

He said, "What are you saying? You will destroy my life. If I make this a condition, then I cannot love."

"But," I told him, "this is the same as you are doing. Meditation is just like love, you have to know it first. God is just like love.

That's why Jesus says that God is love. It is just like love. First one has to experience."

A logical mind can be closed, and so logically that he will never feel that he has closed his own doors to all the possibilities for all growth. So inference, *anuman*, means thinking in such a way that growth is helped. Then it can become a source of right-knowledge.

And the third is the most beautiful, and nowhere else has it been made a source of right-knowledge: the words of the awakened ones, *agama*. There has been a long controversy about this third source. Patanjali says you can know directly, then it is okay. You can infer rightly, then too you are on the right path and you will reach the source.

But there are a few things you cannot even infer, and you have not known. But you are not the first on this earth, you are not the first seeker. Millions have been seeking for millions of ages, and not only on this planet but on other planets also. The search is eternal, and many have arrived. They have reached the goal, they have entered the temple. Their words are also a source of right-knowledge.

Agama means the words of those who have known. Buddha says something or Jesus says something: we don't know what he is saying, we have not experienced that, so we have no way of judging it. We don't know what and how to infer rightly through his words. And the words are contradictory so you can infer anything you like.

There are a few who think Jesus was neurotic. Western psychiatrists have been trying to prove that he was neurotic, he was a maniac. These people claim that in saying, "I am the son of God, and the *only* son" he was mad, an egomaniac, neurotic. It can be proved that he was neurotic because there are many neurotic people who claim such things. You can find them; in madhouses there are many such people.

It happened once in Baghdad. Caliph Omar was the king, and one man declared on the streets of Baghdad, "I am the *paigambara,* I am the messenger, I am the prophet. And now Mohammed is canceled because I am here. I am the last word, the last message from the divine. And now there is no need for Mohammed, he is just out of date. He was the messenger up to now but now I have come. Now you can forget Mohammed."

It was not a Hindu country. Hindus can tolerate everything; no one has tolerated like the Hindus. They can tolerate everything because they say, "Unless we know exactly we cannot say yes, we cannot say no. He may be the messenger, who knows?"

But Mohammedans are different; they are very dogmatic. They cannot tolerate. So Caliph Omar, having caught the new prophet, threw him in jail and told him, "Twenty-four hours are being given to you. Reconsider. And if you say you are not the prophet, that Mohammed is the prophet, then you will be released. If you insist in your madness, then after twenty-four hours I will come to the jail and you will be killed."

The man laughed. He said, "Look! This is written in the scripture – that prophets will always be treated like this, as you are treating me." He was logical. Mohammed himself was treated like that, so this was nothing new. The man said to Omar, "This is nothing new. This is how things are naturally going to be. And I am not in any position to reconsider. I am not the authority, I am just the messenger. Only God can change. In twenty-four hours you can come, you will find me the same. Only he can change who has appointed me."

While this talk was going on another madman, who was chained to a pillar, started laughing. So Omar asked, "Why are you laughing?"

He said, "This man is absolutely wrong. I never appointed him! I cannot allow this. After Mohammed I have not sent any messenger."

In every madhouse these people are there, and it can be proved that Jesus is a similar case.

Words are so contradictory and illogical, and every person who has known is compelled to speak contradictorily, paradoxically, because the truth is such that it can be expressed only through paradoxes. Their statements are not clear, they are mysterious. And you can conclude anything out of them if you infer. You infer, your mind is there. The inference is going to be *your* inference. So Patanjali says there is a third source.

You don't know. If you know directly, then there is no question, then there is no need for any other source. If you have direct cognition, then there is no need for inference or for the words of the enlightened ones; you yourself have become enlightened. Then you can drop the other two sources. Then inference, but the inference will be yours. If you are mad then your inference will be mad. But if this has not happened, then the third source is worth trying – the words of the enlightened ones.

You cannot prove them, you cannot disprove them. You can only have trust, and that trust is hypothetical; it is very scientific. In science also you cannot proceed without a hypothesis. But a hypothesis is not belief; it is just a working arrangement. A hypothesis is just a direction, you will have to experiment. And if the experiment proves right then the hypothesis becomes a theory. If the experiment goes wrong then the hypothesis is discarded. The words of the enlightened ones are to be taken on trust, as a hypothesis. Then work them out in your life. If they prove true, then the hypothesis has become a faith, if they prove false then the hypothesis has to be discarded.

You go to Buddha. He will say, "Wait! Be patient, meditate, and for two years don't ask any question." This you have to take on trust, there is no other way.

You can think, "This man may be just deceiving me. Then two years of my life are wasted. If after two years it is proved that this man was just hocus-pocus, just a deceiver or self-deceived, in an illusion that he has become enlightened, then my two years are wasted." But there is no other way. You have to take the risk. And if you remain there without trusting Buddha, these two years will be useless because unless you trust you cannot work. The work is so intense that only if you have trust can you move wholly into it, totally into it. If you don't have trust then you go on withholding something, and that withholding will not allow you to experience what Buddha is indicating.

There is risk, but life itself is risk. For a higher life there will be higher risks. You move on a dangerous path. But remember, there is only one error in life, and that is not moving at all; that is, just sitting afraid that if you move something may go wrong, so it is better to wait and sit. This is the only error. You will not be in danger but no growth will be possible.

Patanjali says there are things which you do not know, there are things which your logic cannot infer; you have to take on trust. Because of this third source, the guru, the master, becomes a necessity – someone who knows. And you have to take the risk, and I say it is a risk because there is no guarantee. The whole thing may prove just a waste, but it is better to take the risk because even if it is proved to be a waste, you have learned much. Now no other person will be able to deceive you so easily. At least you have learned this much.

If you move with trust, if you move totally, follow a buddha like a shadow, things may start happening because they have happened to the person. They have happened to this Gautam Buddha, to Jesus, to Mahavira, and they know the path they have traveled. If you argue with them you will be the loser. They cannot be the losers, they will simply leave you aside.

In this century this has happened with Gurdjieff. So many people were attracted to him, but he would create such a situation for the new disciples that unless they could trust totally, unless they could trust even in absurdities, they would have to leave immediately. And those absurdities were planned. Gurdjieff would go on lying. In the morning he would say something, in the afternoon something else. And you were not to ask! He would shatter your logical mind completely.

In the morning he would say, "Dig this ditch. And this is a must! By the evening this must be complete." The whole day you would spend digging it. You exerted, you were tired, you were perspiring, you had not eaten, and by evening he would come and say, "Throw the mud back in the ditch. And before you go to bed it has to be completed."

Now even an ordinary mind will say, "What do you mean? I have wasted the whole day. And I was thinking it was something very necessary, by the evening it has to be completed and now you say, 'Throw the mud back!'"

If you asked such a thing Gurdjieff would say, "Simply leave! Go! I am not for you, you are not for me."

The ditch or the digging was not the thing. What he was testing was whether you could trust him even when he was absurd. And once he knew that you could trust him and you could move with him wherever he led, only then real things would follow. Then the test was over, you had been examined and found to be authentic, a real seeker who could work and who could trust. And then real things could happen to you, never before.

Patanjali is a master, and he knows this third source very well through his own experience with thousands and thousands of disciples. He must have worked with many, many disciples and seekers; only then is it possible to write such a treatise as the *Yoga Sutras*. They are not by a thinker, they are by one who has experimented with many types of minds and who has penetrated with many, many layers of minds, every type of person who has worked. He makes this the third source: the words of the awakened ones.

The second sutra:

Wrong-knowledge is a false conception not
corresponding to the thing as it is.

Now some definitions which will be helpful later on: The definition of *viparyaya,* wrong-knowledge. *Wrong-knowledge is a false*
conception of something *not corresponding to the thing as it is.*
We all have a big burden of wrong-knowledge because before we
encounter a fact we are already prejudiced.

If you are a Hindu and someone is introduced to you and it
is said that he is a Mohammedan, immediately you have taken a
wrong attitude that this man must be wrong. If you are a Christian
and someone is introduced as a Jew you are *not* going to "dig" this
man, you are not going to be open to this particular man. Just by
saying "a Jew" your prejudice has come in; you have already known
this man. Now there is no need, you know what type of man this is,
he is a Jew.

You have a preconception, a prejudiced mind, and this prejudiced
mind gives you wrong-knowledge. All Jews are not bad; neither are
all Christians good nor are all Mohammedans bad; neither are all
Hindus good. Really, goodness and badness don't belong to any race,
they belong to persons, individuals. There may be bad Mohammedans, bad Hindus, good Mohammedans, good Hindus. Goodness
and badness do not belong to any nation, to any race, to any culture,
they belong to individuals, personalities. But it's difficult to face a
person without any prejudice; and you will have a revelation.

Once it happened to me while I was traveling...

I entered my compartment on a train. Many people had come to
see me off, so the person who was in the compartment, another
passenger, immediately touched my feet and said, "You must be a
great saint. So many persons have come to see you off."

So I told this man, "I am a Mohammedan. I may be a great saint
but I am a Mohammedan."

He felt shocked! He had touched a Mohammedan's feet and he
was a brahmin! He started perspiring, he was nervous. He looked
again and he said, "No, you are joking." Just to console himself he
said, "You are joking."

"I am not joking. Why should I joke? You should have inquired before you touched my feet!"

Then we were both together in the compartment. Again and again he would look at me and would take a long, deep breath. He must have been thinking to go and take a bath! But he was not encountering me. I was there, and he was concerned with a concept of "Mohammedan." And he was a brahmin; he had become impure by touching me.

Nobody encounters things, persons, as they are – you have a prejudice. These prejudices create *viparyaya*, these prejudices create wrong-knowledge. Whatsoever you think, if you have not come freshly upon the fact, it is going to be wrong. Don't bring your past, don't bring your prejudices. Put aside your mind and encounter the fact. Just see whatsoever there is to be seen. Don't project.

We go on projecting. Our mind is just completely filled and fixed from the very childhood. Everything has been given to us ready made, and through that ready-made knowledge our whole life becomes an illusion. You never meet a real person, you never see a real flower. Just by hearing "This is a rose" you say "Beautiful!" mechanically. You have not felt the beauty, you have not sensed the beauty, you have not touched *this* flower. Just "rose is beautiful" is in your mind; the moment you hear "rose" the mind projects and says "It is beautiful."

You may believe that you have come to feel that the rose is beautiful; this is not so. This is false. Just look. That's why children come to things more deeply than grown-up people, because they don't know names. They are not yet prejudiced. If a rose is beautiful only then will it be beautiful; not all roses are beautiful. Children come near to things, their eyes are fresh. They see things as they are because they don't know how to project anything.

But we are always in a hurry to make them grown-ups, to make them adults. We are filling their minds with knowledge, information. This is one of the most recent discoveries of psychologists: that when children enter school they have more intelligence than when they leave the university. The latest findings prove that when children enter the first grade, they have more intelligence, and they will have less and less intelligence as they grow in knowledge. And by the time they become bachelors and masters and doctors, they are finished. When they come back with a doctor's degree, a Ph.D., they have left their intelligence somewhere in the university. They are dead, filled with knowledge, crammed with knowledge, but this knowledge is just false, a prejudice about everything. Now they cannot feel things directly, they cannot feel live persons directly, they cannot live directly. Everything has become verbal, wordy. It is not real now, it has become mental.

Wrong-knowledge is a false conception not corresponding to the thing as it is.

Put aside your prejudices, knowledge, conceptions, pre-formulated information and look fresh, become a child again. And this has to be done moment to moment because every moment you are gathering.

One of the oldest Yoga aphorisms is: Die every moment so you can be reborn every moment. Die every moment to the past, throw off all the dust that you have collected and look afresh. But this has to be done continuously because next moment the dust has gathered again.

Nan-in was in search of a Zen master when he was a seeker. He lived with his master for many years, and then the master said, "Everything is okay. You have almost achieved."

But he said "almost," so Nan-in said, "What do you mean?"

The master said, "I will have to send you to another master for a few days. That will do the last finishing touch." Nan-in was very excited. He said, "Send me immediately!" A letter was given to him. And he was excited; he thought he was being sent to someone who was a greater master than his own. But when he reached to the man he was a nobody, just a keeper of an inn, a doorkeeper of an inn.

He felt very disappointed and he thought, "This must be some sort of joke. This man is going to be my last master? He is going to give me the finishing touch?" But he had come, so he thought, "It is better to be here for a few days at least to rest, then I will go back. It was a long journey." So he said to the innkeeper, "My master has given this letter."

The innkeeper said, "But I cannot read, so you can keep your letter; it is not needed. And you can be here."

Nan-in said, "But I have been sent to learn something from you."

The innkeeper said, "I am just an innkeeper. I am not a master, I am not a teacher. There must have been some misunderstanding.

You may have come to a wrong person. I am just an innkeeper. I cannot teach; I don't know anything. But since you have come you can just watch me. That may be helpful. You rest and watch."

But there was nothing to watch. In the morning he would open the door of the inn. Then guests would come and he would clean their things – the pots, the utensils and everything – and he would serve. And in the night again, when everybody had gone and the guests had gone to sleep to their beds, he would clean things again, pots, utensils, everything. And in the morning, again the same.

By the third day Nan-in was bored. And he said, "There is nothing to watch. You go on cleaning utensils, you go on doing ordinary work, so I must leave." The innkeeper laughed, but said nothing.

Nan-in went back. He was very angry with his master and said, "Why? Why was I sent for such a long journey? It was tedious, and the man was just an innkeeper. And he didn't teach me anything, and he simply said, 'Watch' – and there was nothing to watch."

But the master said, "Still, you were there for three, four days. Even if there was nothing to watch, you must have watched. What were you doing?"

So he said, "I was watching! In the night he would clean the utensils, pots, put everything there, and in the morning he was again cleaning."

The master said, "This! This is the teaching! This is what you were sent for! He had cleaned those pots in the night, but in the morning he was again cleaning those clean pots. What does it mean? Because even in the night, when nothing had happened, they had become unclean again, some dust had settled again. So you may be pure – now you are – you may be innocent, but every moment you have to continue cleaning. You may not do anything, still you become impure just by the passage of time. Moment by moment, just with the passage of time, not doing anything, just sitting under a tree, you become unclean. And that uncleanliness is not because you were doing something bad or something wrong, it happens just through the passage of time. Dust collects, so you go on cleaning. And this is the last touch – because I feel you have become proud that you are pure and now you are not aware of a constant effort to clean."

Moment to moment one has to die and be reborn again. Only then are you freed from wrong-knowledge.

The third sutra:

An image conjured up by words without any
substance behind it is vikalpa, imagination.

Imagination is just through words, verbal structures. You create a thing – it is not there, it is not a reality, but you create it through your mental images. And you can create it to such an extent that you yourself become deceived by it and you think it is real. This happens in hypnosis. Hypnotize a person and say anything; he conjures up the image and that image becomes real. You can do it, you are doing it in many ways.

One of the most famous Swedish actresses, Greta Garbo, has written a memoir. She was an ordinary girl, just a homely, ordinary girl, very poor, and working in a barber shop. Just for a few pennies she would put lather on the customers' faces. She did this for three years.

One day, an American film director was in that barber shop and she was putting soap on his face, and just the way Americans are – he may not have even meant it – he simply looked in the mirror at the reflection of the girl, and said, "How beautiful!" And Greta Garbo was born that very moment.

She writes that suddenly she became different. She had never thought herself beautiful, she couldn't conceive of it. And she had never heard anybody saying that she was beautiful. For the first time she also looked in the mirror and the face was different, this man had made her beautiful. And her whole life changed. She followed the man and became one of the most famous film actresses.

What happened? Just hypnosis, hypnosis through a word *beautiful*, worked. It works, it becomes chemical. Everybody believes something about himself: that belief becomes reality because that belief starts working on you.

Imagination is a force, but it is a conjured-up force, an imagined force. You can use it and you can be used by it. If you can use it, it will be helpful, but if you are used by it, it is fatal, it is dangerous. Imagination can become madness any moment. Imagination can be helpful if through it you create a situation for your inner growth and crystallization. But it is through words, a conjured-up thing.

For human beings words, language, verbal constructions have become so significant that now nothing is more significant. If someone suddenly says, "Fire!" the word *fire* will change you immediately. There may be no fire... You will stop listening to me. There will be no effort to stop; suddenly you will stop listening to me, you will start running here and there. The word *fire* has taken your imagination.

In that way you are influenced by words. The people in the advertisement business know what words to use to conjure up images. Through those words they catch you, they catch the whole market. There are many such words. They go on changing with the fashions.

In the past few years *new* is the word. So everything you see in the advertisements is new – a "new" Lux soap. Lux soap won't do; the new appeals immediately. Everybody is for the new. Everybody is searching for the new, something new, because everybody is bored with the old. So anything new has appeal. That may not be better than the old – it may be worse – but just the word *new* opens vistas in the mind.

These words and their influence have to be understood deeply. A person who is in search of the truth must be aware of the influence of words. Politicians and advertising people are using words, and they can create through words, they can capture your imagination so much that you can even stake your life; you can throw your life away just for words.

What are these? – "Nation," "the national flag" – just words. "Hinduism"... You can say "Hinduism is in danger" and suddenly many people are ready to do something or even to die – just a few words! "Our nation is insulted": what is "our nation"? – just words. A flag is nothing but a piece of cloth, but a whole nation can die for the flag because someone has insulted the flag, lowered it. What nonsense goes on in this world because of words! Words are dangerous, they have deep sources of influence within you. They trigger something in you and you can be captured.

Patanjali says imagination has to be understood, because on the path of meditation words have to be dropped so that influence by others can be dropped. Remember, words are taught by others, you are not born with words. They are taught to you and through words, many prejudices are taught. Through words religion, through words myths, everything is fed to you through words. The word is the medium, the vehicle of culture, society, information.

You cannot excite animals to fight for a nation. You cannot excite them because they don't know what a "nation" is. That's why there are no wars. In the animal kingdom there are no wars, no flags, no temples, no mosques. And if animals can look at us, they are bound to think that man has some obsession with words, because wars go on around them, millions are killed just because of words.

Someone is a Jew, kill him – just the word *Jew*. Change the label, he becomes a Christian, and then there is no need to kill. But he is not ready to change the label. He will say, "I would rather be killed but I cannot change my label. I am a Jew." He is also adamant, others are also adamant. But just words!

Jean-Paul Sartre has written his autobiography and he has given it the title *Words*. It is beautiful, because as far as mind is concerned the whole autobiography of *any* mind consists of words and nothing else. And Patanjali says one has to be aware of this, because on the path of meditation words have to be left behind. Nations, religions, scriptures, languages have to be left behind and man has to become innocent, freed of words. When you are free of words there will be no imagination, and when there is no imagination you can face truth. Otherwise you will go on creating.

If you go to meet God, you must meet him without any words. If you have some words, he may not fit and suit your idea. Because if a Hindu thinks God has one thousand hands and if God comes with only two hands, he will reject: "You are not a God at all. With only two hands? God has a thousand hands. Show me your other hands, only then can I believe."

I have heard...

One of the most beautiful persons of this past century was Sai Baba of Shirdi. Sai Baba was a Mohammedan. Really, no one knows whether he was a Mohammedan or a Hindu, but he lived in a mosque so it was believed that he was a Mohammedan. He had a friend and a follower who was a Hindu who loved, respected, had much faith in Sai Baba. Every day he would come for his *darshan*, and unless he saw him he would not leave. Sometimes it would happen that for the whole day he would have to wait, but he would not go without seeing him, and he would not take food unless he had seen Sai Baba.

Once it happened that the whole day passed, there was a big gathering and much crowding; he couldn't enter. When everybody had gone, just in the night he reached Sai Baba and touched his feet.

Sai Baba said to him, "Why do you wait unnecessarily? There is no need to see me here, I can come there. And drop this; from tomorrow, now I will come. You will see me every day before you take your food."

The disciple was very happy. So the next day he waited and waited: nothing happened. Really, many things happened, but nothing happened according to his conception. By the evening he was very angry. He had not eaten and Sai Baba had not appeared, so he went again. He said, "You promise and you don't fulfill?"

Sai Baba said, "But I appeared thrice, not even once. First time I came I was a beggar, and you said to me, 'Move away. Don't come here.' The second time I came as an old woman, and you just wouldn't look at me; you closed your eyes" – because the disciple had the habit of not seeing women; he was practicing not seeing women, so he closed his eyes. Sai Baba said, "I had come, but what do you expect? Should I enter your closed eyes? I was standing there but you closed your eyes. The moment you saw me you closed the eyes. Then the third time I came as a dog, and you wouldn't allow me in. You were standing at the door with a stick."

And these three things had happened. And these things have been happening to the whole humanity. The divine comes in many forms but you have a prejudice; you have a pre-formulated conception, you cannot see. He must appear according to you, and he never appears according to you, and he will never appear according to you. You cannot be the rule for him and you cannot put any conditions.

When all imagination falls away, only then truth appears. Otherwise imagination goes on making conditions and truth cannot appear. Only in a naked mind, in a nude, empty mind, truth appears, because you cannot distort it.

The fourth sutra:

The modification of the mind which is based
on the absence of any content in it is sleep.

This is the definition of sleep, the fourth modification of the mind: when there is no content. Mind is always with content, except in sleep. Something or other is there. Some thought is moving, some passion is moving, some desire is moving, some memory, some future

imagination, some word, something is moving. Something is continuously there. Only when you are fast asleep, deeply asleep, content
stops, mind disappears and you are in yourself without any content.

This has to be remembered because this is going to be the state
of *samadhi* also, with only one difference: you will be aware. In sleep
you are unaware, mind goes completely to non-existence. You are
alone, left alone with no thought, just your being. But you are not
aware. Mind is not there to disturb you, but you are not aware; otherwise sleep can become enlightenment.

Contentless consciousness is there, but the consciousness is not
alert. It is hidden, just in a seed. In *samadhi* the seed is broken, the
consciousness becomes alert. And when consciousness is alert and
there is no content, this is the goal. Sleep with awareness is the goal.

This is the fourth modification of the mind – sleep. But that goal,
sleep with awareness, is not a modification of the mind, it is beyond
mind. Awareness is beyond mind. If you can join sleep and awareness together, you have become enlightened. But it is difficult
because even when we are awake in the day, we are not alert. Even
when we are awake, we are not awake; the word is false. When we
sleep, how can we be awake, when even when we are awake, we are
not awake.

So one has to start in the day, when you are awake. You have to
be more awake, more and more intensely awake. And then you have
to try with dreams: in dreams you have to be alert. Only if you succeed with the waking state, then with the dreaming state, will you be
able to succeed with the third state, of sleep.

Try first walking on the street: try to be aware. Don't just go on
walking automatically, mechanically. Be alert of every movement, of
every breath that you take – exhale, inhale – be alert. Of every eye
movement you are doing, of every person you look at, be alert.
Whatever you are doing, be alert and do it with alertness.

Then at night, while you are falling asleep, try to remain alert.
The last phase of the day will be passing, memories will be floating –
remain alert and try to fall asleep with alertness. It will be difficult,
but if you try, within a few weeks you will have a glimpse: you are
asleep and alert. If you can manage even for a single moment, it is
so beautiful, it is so bliss-filled that you will never be the same again.

Then you will not say that sleep is just wasting time. It can
become the most precious *sadhana,* because when the waking state

goes and the sleeping starts there is a change, a change of gears inside. It is just like a change of gears in a car. When you change gears from one gear to another, for a single moment between these two there is a neutral gear, there is no gear. That moment of neutrality is very significant.

The same happens in the mind. When from waking you move into sleep, there is a moment when you are neither awake nor asleep. In that moment there is no gear, the mechanism is not functioning. Your automatic personality is nullified in that moment. In that moment your old habits will not force you in a certain pattern. In that moment you can escape and become alert.

In India this moment has been called *sandhya*, the moment in between. There are two *sandhyas*, two in-between moments: one in the night when you go from waking to sleep, and the other in the morning when you again move from sleep to waking. Hindus have called these two the moments of prayerfulness, *sandhyakal*, the period in between, because then for a single moment your personality is not there. In that single moment you are pure, innocent. If in that moment you can become alert, your whole life will change. You will have a base for transformation.

Then try to be alert in the dream state. There are methods for how to be alert in a dream state. If you want to try, first try in the waking state. When you succeed in the waking, then you will be able to succeed in the dreaming because dreaming is deeper, more effort will be needed. And it is also difficult because what to do in a dream and how to do it?

For the dreaming state, Gurdjieff developed a beautiful method. It is one of the old Tibetan methods, and Tibetan seekers have worked very deeply into the dreamworld.

The method is: just when falling into sleep try to remember one thing, any one thing, perhaps just a roseflower. Just visualize a roseflower and go on thinking that you will see it in the dream. Visualize it and go on thinking that in the dream, whatsoever the dream, this roseflower must be there. Visualize its color, its scent, everything. Feel it so it will become alive inside you, and with that roseflower fall into sleep.

Within a few days you will be able to bring that flower into your dream. This is a great success, because now you have created at least a part of the dream. Now you are the master. At least one part of the dream, the flower, has come. And the moment you see the flower you will immediately remember, "This is a dream." Nothing else is needed. The flower and, "This is a dream" have become associated because you have created the flower in the dream. And you were continuously thinking for this flower to appear in the dream and the flower has appeared. Immediately you will recognize, "This is a dream," and the whole quality of the dream will change, the flower-dream and everything around the dream. You have become alert.

Then you can enjoy the dream in a new way, just like a film. And then if you want to stop the dream you can simply stop, put it off. But that will take a little more time and more practice. Then you can create your own dreams. There is no need to be a victim of dreams: you can create your own dreams, you can live your own dreams. You can have a theme just before you fall into sleep, you can direct your dreams just like a film director and you can create a theme out of it.

Tibetans have used dream creations because through dream creation you can change your total mind, the structure. And when you succeed in dreams then you can succeed in sleep. But there is no technique for sleep because there is no content. A technique can work only with content. Because there is no content, no technique can help. But through dream you will learn to be aware and that awareness can be carried on into sleep.

The last sutra:

Memory is the calling up of past experiences.

These are definitions. He is clarifying things so later on you need not get mixed up.

What is memory? – calling up of past experiences. Memory is continuously happening. Whenever you see something, immediately memory comes in and distorts it. You have seen me before. You see me again and immediately memory comes in. If you had seen me five years before, then the picture of five years ago, the past picture, will come into your eyes and fill your eyes, and you will see me through that picture.

That's why if you have not seen your friend for many days, the moment you see him you immediately say, "You are looking very thin," or "You are looking very unhealthy," or "You have gained weight." Immediately! Why? – because you are comparing; the memory has come in. The man himself is not aware that he has gotten fat or he has become thin, but you become aware because immediately you can compare. The past, the last picture comes in, and immediately you can compare.

This memory is continuously there, being projected on everything you see. This past memory has to be dropped. It should not be a constant interference in your knowing because it doesn't allow you to know the new. You always know in the pattern of the old. It doesn't allow you to feel the new, it makes everything old and rotten. Because of this memory, everybody is bored; the whole humanity is bored. Look at anybody's face – he is bored, bored to death. There is nothing new, no ecstasy.

Why are children so ecstatic? You cannot imagine how this ecstasy is happening for such simple things. Just a few colored stones on the beach and they start dancing. What is happening to them? Why can't you dance? – because you know those are just stones, your memory is there. For those children there is no memory, those stones are a new phenomenon, as if they have reached to the moon.

I was reading that when the first man reached the moon there was excitement all over the world. And everybody was looking at their TV's – but within fifteen minutes everybody was bored, finished: "What to do now? The man is walking on the moon." After just fifteen minutes – and this dream had taken millions of years to reach there – and now nobody was interested in what was happening.

Everything becomes old. Immediately it becomes memory, it becomes old. If you can, drop your memories, and dropping doesn't mean that you cease to remember, dropping only means dropping this constant interference. When you need it you can pull it back into focus. When you don't need it just let it be there, silent, not continuously coming.

The past, if continuously present, will not allow the present to be. And if you miss the present you miss all.

Enough for today.

the purity of yoga

The first question:

Osho,
You said that Patanjali's Yoga is an exact science,
absolutely logical, in which the result is as certain as two
plus two make four. If the attainment of the unknown
and infinite can be reduced to mere logic, is it not true
and at the same time absurd that the infinite
phenomenon is within the orbit of the finite mind?

It looks absurd, it looks illogical, but existence is absurd and existence is illogical. The sky is infinite, but it can be reflected in a very tiny pool; the infinite sky can be reflected in a small mirror. Of course the whole of it will not be reflected, it cannot be reflected. But the part is also the whole and the part also belongs to the sky.

The human mind is just a mirror. If it is pure then the infinite can have the reflection in it. The reflection will not be the infinite. It will be just a part, a glimpse, but that glimpse becomes the door. Then, by and by, you can leave the mirror behind and enter into the infinite, leave the reflection behind and enter into the real.

Out of your window, the small frame of the window is the infinite sky. You can look through the window. You will not see the whole sky, of course, but whatsoever you see is the sky. The only thing to remember is, don't think that whatsoever you have seen is the infinite. It may be *of* the infinite, it is not the infinite. So whatsoever the human mind can conceive may be divine, but it is just a part of it, a glimpse. If you continuously remember that, then there is no fallacy. Then, by and by, destroy the frame. By and by, destroy the mind completely so the mirror is no longer there and you are freed from the reflection and you enter the reality.

On the surface it looks absurd. How, in such a tiny mind, can there be any contact with the eternal, with the infinite, with the endless? A second thing has also to be understood. This tiny mind is also not really tiny, because it is also part of the infinite. It looks tiny because of you, it looks finite because of you. You have created the boundaries. The boundaries are false. Even your tiny mind belongs to the infinite, it is part of it.

There are many things to be understood. One of the most paradoxical things about the infinite is that the part is always equal to the whole. You cannot divide the infinite. All divisions are false. It may be utilitarian to divide it: I can say that the sky on my house, on my terrace, is *my* sky, just as India says that the sky on the Indian continent is Indian sky. What do you mean? You cannot divide the sky. It cannot be Indian or Chinese, it is an undivided expanse. It begins nowhere, it ends nowhere.

This has also happened with the mind. You call it your mind; that "your" is false. The mind is part of the infinite. Just as matter is part of the infinite, mind is part of the infinite. Your soul is also part of the infinite. When the "my" is lost you are the infinite. So if you appear finite, it is an illusion.

Finiteness is not a reality; finiteness is just a conception, an illusion. Because of your conception you are confined in it. And whatsoever you think, you become. Buddha has said – and he was repeating it continuously for forty years – that whatsoever you think you become. Thinking makes you whatsoever you are. If you are finite, it is a standpoint that you have taken. Drop the standpoint and you become infinite.

The whole process of Yoga is how to drop the frame, how to destroy the mirror, how to move from the reflection to the reality, how to go beyond the boundaries. Boundaries are self-created, they are not really there. They are just thoughts. That's why, whenever there is no thought in the mind, you are not. A thoughtless mind is egoless, a thoughtless mind is boundless, a thoughtless mind is already the infinite. If even for a single moment there is no thought, you are the infinite, because without thought there can be no boundary. Without thought you disappear and the divine descends.

To be in thought is to be human, to be below thought is to be animal, to be beyond thought is to be divine. But the logical mind will raise questions, the logical mind will say, "How can the part be equal to the whole? The part must be less than the whole. It cannot be the equal."

Ouspensky writes in *Tertium Organum,* one of the best, one of the few great books in the world, that not only can the part be the equal to the whole, it can be even greater than the whole. But he calls it a higher mathematics. That mathematics belongs to the Upanishads. In the *Ishavasya Upanishad* it is said, "You can take out the whole from the whole, and still the whole remains behind. You can put the whole into the whole, and still the whole remains the whole." It is absurd. If you like to call it absurd you can call it absurd. But really, it is a higher mathematics where boundaries are lost and the drop becomes the ocean and the ocean is nothing but a drop.

Logic raises questions, it goes on raising them. That is the nature of the logical mind, to raise questions. And if you go on following those questions you can go on ad infinitum. Put aside the mind, its logic, its reasoning, and for a few moments try to be without thought. If you can achieve that state of non-thought even for a single moment you will come to realize that the part is equal to the whole, because suddenly you will see all the boundaries have disappeared. They were dream boundaries. All the divisions have disappeared, and you and the whole have become one.

This can be an experience. This cannot be a logical inference. Then when I say that Patanjali is logical, what do I mean? In the conclusions, nobody can be logical as far as the inner, the spiritual, the ultimate experience is concerned. But on the path, you can be logical. As far as the ultimate result of Yoga is concerned, Patanjali also cannot be logical; nobody can be. But to reach that goal you can follow a logical path.

In that sense Patanjali is logical and rational, mathematical,

scientific. He does not ask any faith. He asks only for the courage
to experiment, courage to move, courage to take a jump into the
unknown. He does not say, "Believe and then you will experience."
He says, "Experience and then you will believe." And he has made a
structure of how to proceed step by step. His path is not haphazard;
it is not like a labyrinth, it is like a superhighway. Everything is clear
and the shortest possible route. But you have to follow it in every
detail, otherwise you will move off the path and into the wilderness.

That's why I say he is logical, and you will see how he is logical.
He starts from the body because you are rooted in the body. He
starts and works with your breathing because your breathing is your
life. First he works on the body, then he works on the *prana* – the
second layer of existence – your breathing; then he starts working
on thoughts.

There are many methods which start directly with the thoughts.
They are not so logical and scientific because the man you are
working with is rooted in the body. He is a *soma,* a body. A scientific
approach must start with the body. Your body must be changed first.
When your body changes, then your breathing can be changed. When
your breathing changes, then your thoughts can be changed. And
when your thoughts change then you can be changed.

You may not have observed that you are a close-knit system of
many layers. When you are running your breathing changes because
more oxygen is needed, and when your breathing changes your
thoughts immediately change.

In Tibet they say if you are angry, then just run. Do two or three
rounds of your house, and then come back and see where your
anger has gone because if you run fast your breathing changes; if
your breathing changes your thought pattern cannot remain the
same, it has to change.

There is no need to run: you can simply take five deep breaths –
exhale, inhale – and see where your anger has gone. It is difficult to
change anger directly. It is easier to change the body, then the
breathing, then the anger. This is a scientific process. That is why I
say that Patanjali is scientific. Nobody else has been so scientific.

If you go to Buddha he will say, "Drop anger." Patanjali will never
say that. He will say if you have anger, that means you have a
breathing pattern which helps anger, and unless that breathing pattern is changed you cannot drop anger. You may do, with struggle,

but that is not going to help, or it may take a very long time, unnecessary time. So he will watch your breathing pattern, the breathing rhythm, and if you have a certain breathing rhythm that means you have a certain body posture for it.

The grossest is the body and the subtlest is the mind. Don't start from the subtle because it will be more difficult. It is vague, you cannot grasp it. Start with the body. That's why Patanjali starts with body postures.

You may not have observed, because you are so unalert in life, that whenever you have a certain mood in the mind you have a certain body posture associated with it. If you are angry, can you sit relaxed? – impossible. If you are angry your body posture will change, if you are attentive then your body posture will change, if you are sleepy your body posture will change.

If you are completely silent you will sit buddha-like, you will walk buddha-like. If you walk buddha-like, you will feel a certain silence merging within your heart. A certain silent bridge is being created by your buddha-like walk. Just sit under a tree like a buddha. Just sit, just the body: suddenly you will see that your breathing is changing – it is more relaxed, it is more harmonious. When the breathing is harmonious and relaxed, you will feel the mind is less tense. There are fewer thoughts, fewer clouds, more space, more sky. You will feel a silence in and out, flowing.

Hence I say Patanjali is scientific. If you want to change the body posture, Patanjali will say change your food habits, because every food habit creates subtle body postures. If you are an eater of meat you cannot sit buddha-like. If you are non-vegetarian your posture will be different than if you are a vegetarian; your postures will be different because the body is built by your food. It is not an accident. Whatsoever you are putting in the body, the body will reflect it.

So for Patanjali vegetarianism is not a moralist cult, it is a scientific method. When you eat meat you are not only taking food, you are allowing a certain animal from which the meat has come to enter in you. The meat was part of a particular body; the meat was part of a particular instinct pattern. The meat was the animal just a few hours before, and that meat carries all the impressions of the animal, all the habits of the animal. When you are eating meat your many attitudes will be affected by it.

If you are sensitive you can become aware that whenever you eat certain things, certain changes immediately take place. You can drink alcohol and then you do not remain the same, immediately a new personality comes in. Alcohol cannot create a personality but it changes your body pattern, the body chemistry is changed. With the change of the body chemistry the mind has to change its pattern, and when the mind changes its pattern a new personality comes in.

I have heard...

One of the oldest Chinese parables is that once a bottle of whisky fell down from a table, just by accident – a cat might have jumped. The bottle was broken and the whisky was spilled all over the floor. In the night three mice lapped at the whisky. One mouse immediately said, "Now I am going to the king, to the palace, to put him right in his place."

The other said, "I am not worried about kings. I myself am going to be the emperor of the whole earth."

And the third said, "Do whatsoever you like, you fellows. I am going upstairs to make love to the cat."

The whole personality has changed – a mouse thinking of making love to a cat? It can happen, it happens every day. Whatsoever you eat changes you, whatsoever you drink changes you because body is a great part; you are ninety percent your bodies.

Patanjali is scientific because he takes note of everything – the food, the posture, the way you sleep, the way you get up in the morning, when you get up in the morning, when you go to sleep. He takes note of everything so that your body becomes a situation for something higher.

Then he takes note of your breathing. If you are sad you have a different rhythm of breathing. Just note it down. Try; you can have a very beautiful experiment. Whenever you are sad just watch your breath; watch how much time you take in inhalation and then how much time you take in exhalation. Just note it down. Just count numbers inside: one, two, three, four, five... You count to five and the inhalation is over. Then you count – it comes to ten and the exhalation is over. Just watch it minutely so you can come to know the ratio. Then whenever you feel happy immediately try that sad pattern – five, ten – and the happiness will disappear.

The reverse is also true. Whenever you feel happy note down how you are breathing, and whenever you feel sad try that pattern. Immediately, sadness will disappear, because mind cannot exist in a vacuum. It exists in a system, and breathing is the deepest system for the mind.

Breath is thought. If you stop breathing, immediately thoughts stop. Try it for a second. Stop the breathing. Immediately there is a break in the thinking process; the process is broken. Thinking is the invisible part of the visible breathing.

That's what I mean when I say Patanjali is scientific. He is not a poet. If he says, "Don't eat meat," he is not saying it because eating meat is violence, no. He is saying it because eating meat is self-destructive. There are poets who say to be nonviolent is beautiful; Patanjali says to be nonviolent is to be healthy, to be nonviolent is to be selfish. You are not having compassion on somebody else, you are having compassion on yourself.

He is concerned with you – and the transformation. And you cannot change things just by thinking about change, you have to create the situation. Otherwise, all over the world love has been taught, but love exists nowhere because the situation doesn't exist. How can you be loving if you are a meat-eater? If you are eating meat, the violence is there. And with such a deep violence how can you be loving? Your love will be just false. Or, it may be just a form of hate.

There is an old Indian tale:

A Christian missionary was passing through a forest. Of course he believed in love, so he was not carrying a gun. Suddenly he saw a lion approaching. He became afraid. He started to think, "Now the gospel of love won't do. It would have been wise if I had a gun."

But something had to be done, and he was in an emergency. Then he remembered somebody has said somewhere that if you run then the lion will follow you, and within minutes you will be caught and dead. But if you stare into the eyes of the lion then there is some possibility he may get impressed, hypnotized. He may change his mind. And there are stories that many times lions have changed their minds, they have slunk away.

So it was worth trying, and there was no use in escaping. The missionary stared. The lion also came near. He also started staring into the eyes of the missionary. For five minutes they were standing face to face, staring into each other's eyes. Then suddenly the missionary saw the miracle. Suddenly the lion put his paws close together and then bent over them in a very prayerful mood, as if he was praying.

This was too much! Even the missionary was not expecting so much – that a lion should start praying. He was happy. But then he thought, "What is to be done now? What should I do?" But by that time he was also hypnotized – not only the lion – so he thought, "It is better to follow the lion."

He also bent over, started praying. Five minutes again passed. Then the lion opened his eyes and said, "Man, what are you doing? I am saying grace, but what are you doing?"

The lion was a religious lion, pious, but just in thought. In deed he was a lion, and he was going to be a lion. He was going to kill the man; he was saying grace.

This is the situation of the whole human phenomenon, the whole of humanity is just pious in thoughts; in deeds, man remains an animal. And this will always be so unless we don't cling to thoughts but create situations in which thoughts change.

Patanjali won't say that it is good to be loving, he will help you to create the situation in which love can flower. This is why I say he is scientific. If you follow him, step by step, you will see many flowerings in you which were inconceivable before, unimaginable. You could not have even dreamed about them. If you change your food, if you change your body posture, if you change your sleeping patterns, if you change ordinary habits, you will see a new person is arising in you. And then there are different changes possible. After one change other changes become possible. Step by step more possibilities open. That's why I say he is logical. He is not a logical philosopher; he is a logical, practical man.

The second question:

Osho,
Yesterday you referred to a Western thinker who started doubting everything that can be doubted, but could not

doubt himself. You said that this is a great achievement
in opening towards the divine. How?

The opening toward higher consciousness means you must
have something indubitable with you – that's what trust means.
You have at least one point which you trust, which you cannot
doubt even if you want to. That's why I said Descartes came to a
point through his logical investigation: "We cannot doubt ourselves.
I cannot doubt that I am, because even to say that I doubt I have to
be there. The very assertion that 'I doubt' proves that I am."

You must have heard the famous dictum of Descartes, "*Cogito,
ergo sum* – I think, therefore I am." Doubting is thinking: I doubt,
therefore I am. But this is just an opening, and Descartes never went
beyond this opening. He again turned back. You can come back
from the very door. He was happy that he had found a center, an
indubitable center, and then he started to work out his philosophy.
So all that he had denied before, he pulled in from the back door:
"Because I am, then there must be a creator who has created me."
And then he went on to heaven and hell, then God and sin and the
whole Christian theology came in from the back door.

He used this as a philosophical inquiry. He was not a yogi; he
was not really in search of his being, he was in search of a theory.
But you can use that as an opening. An opening means you have to
transcend it, you have to go beyond, you have to pass over it, you
have to go through it. You are not to cling to it. If you cling then any
opening will become closed.

It is good to realize: "At least I cannot doubt myself." Then the
right step will be this: "If I cannot doubt myself, if I feel I am, then I
must know who I am." Then it becomes a right inquiry. Then you
move into religion, because when you ask, "Who am I?" you have
asked a fundamental question. Not philosophical – existential.
Nobody else can tell you who you are. Nobody else can give you a
ready-made answer. You will have to search yourself, you will have
to dig it out within yourself.

Just this logical certainty that "I am" is not of much use if you
don't go ahead and ask, "Who am I?" And this is not a question; this
is going to be a quest. A question may lead you into philosophy, a
quest leads you into religion. So if you feel that you don't know
yourself, then don't go to anybody to ask, "Who am I?" Nobody can

answer you. You are there inside, hidden. You have to penetrate to that dimension where you are, encounter yourself.

This is a different type of journey, the inner journey. All our journeys are outer: we are making bridges to reach someone else. This quest means you have to break all the bridges to others. All that you have done without has to be dropped and something new has to be started within. It will be difficult, just because you have become so fixed with the without. You always think of others, you never think of yourself.

This is strange, but no one thinks about himself, he thinks about others. If sometimes you think about yourself it is also in relation to others. It is never pure. It is not simply just about you. Then when you think just about you, thinking will have to be dropped because what can you think? You can think about others; thinking means "about." What can you think about yourself? You will have to drop thinking and you will have to look inside – not thinking but looking, seeing, observing, witnessing. The whole process will change. One has to look for oneself.

Doubt is good. If you doubt, and if you continuously doubt, there is only one rock-like phenomenon which cannot be doubted, and that is your existence. Then a new quest will arise, and that is not a question. You will have to ask, "Who am I?"

His whole life Ramana Maharshi gave only one technique to his disciples. He would say, "Just sit down, close your eyes, and go on asking, 'Who am I? Who am I?' Use it as a mantra." But it is not a mantra. You have not to use it as dead words; it must become an inner penetration: Who am I? Go on asking it. Your mind will answer many times that you are a soul, you are a self, you are divine, but don't listen to these things, these are all borrowed; you have *heard* these things. Put them aside. And if you go on continuously putting the mind aside, one day there is an explosion. The mind explodes and all the borrowed knowledge disappears from you, and for the first time you are face to face with yourself, looking within yourself. This is the opening, and this is the way, and this is the quest.

Ask who you are and don't cling to cheap answers. All answers that are given by others are cheap. The real answer can only come out of you. It is just like a real flower can only come out of the tree itself; you cannot put it onto the tree from the outside. You can, but that will be a dead flower. It may deceive others but it cannot deceive the tree itself. The tree knows, "This is just a dead flower hanging on my branch. And this is just a weight. This is not a happiness, this is just a burden." The tree cannot celebrate it, the tree cannot welcome it.

The tree can welcome only something which comes from the very roots, from its inner being, the innermost core. And when it comes from its innermost core, the flower becomes its soul. And through the flower the tree expresses its dance, its song. Its whole life becomes meaningful. Just like that, the answer will come out of you, out of your roots. Then you will dance it. Then your whole life will become meaningful.

If the answer is given from without it will be just a sign, a dead sign. If it comes from within it will not be a sign, it will be a significance. Remember these two words, *sign* and *significance*. Sign can be given from without, significance can only flower from within. Philosophy works with signs, concepts, words. Religion works with significance; it is not concerned with words, signs or symbols.

But that is going to be an arduous journey for you because nobody can really help, and all the helpers are, in a way, hindrances. If somebody is too patronizing and gives you the answer, he is your enemy. Patanjali is not going to give you the answer, he is only going to indicate to you the path, the way from where your own answer will arise, from where you will encounter the answer.

The great masters have only given methods, they have not given the answer. Philosophers have given answers, but Patanjali, Jesus or Buddha, have not given answers. You ask for answers and they give you methods, they give you techniques. You have to work your answer out yourself through your effort, through your suffering, through your penetration. Only through your *tapascharya* can the answer come, and it can become a significance. Your fulfillment is through it.

The third question:

Osho,
Buddha finally conveyed to Mahakashyapa what he could not convey to anybody else through words. In what category of knowledge – direct, inferential and words of the awakened ones – does it come? What was the message?

First, you ask, "What was the message?" If Buddha could not convey it through words, I also cannot convey it through words. It is not possible.

I will tell you one anecdote...

A disciple came to Mulla Nasruddin and he asked the Mulla, "I have heard that you have the secret, the ultimate secret, the key which can open all the doors of mystery."

Nasruddin said, "Yes, I have got it. But what about it? Why are you asking about it?"

The man fell down at his feet and he said, "I was in search of you, master. If you have the key and the secret, tell it to me."

Nasruddin said, "If it is such a secret, you must understand it cannot be told so easily. You will have to wait."

The disciple asked, "How long?"

Nasruddin said, "That too is not certain. It depends on your patience – three years or thirty years."

The disciple waited. After three years he asked again. Nasruddin said, "If you ask again, then it will take thirty years. Just wait. It is not an ordinary thing, it is the ultimate secret."

Thirty years passed and the disciple said, "Master, now my whole life is wasted. I have not got anything. Now, give me the secret."

Nasruddin said, "There is a condition: you will have to promise me that you will keep it a secret, you will not say it to anybody."

The man said, "I promise you that it will remain a secret until I die. I will not mention it to anyone."

Nasruddin said, "Thank you. This is what my master said to me, and this was my promise to my master. And if you can keep it a secret until death, what do you think? Cannot I keep it a secret?"

If Buddha was silent, I can also be silent about it. There is something which cannot be said. It is not a message, because messages can always be said. And if they cannot be said they cannot be messages. A message is something said, something to be said that can be said. A message is always verbal.

Buddha has not a message, that's why he couldn't say it. There were ten thousand disciples, but only Mahakashyapa got it because he could understand Buddha's silence. That is the secret of the secret: he could understand the silence.

Buddha remained silent under his tree one morning. And he was really going to give a sermon and everybody was waiting. He remained silent. The disciples became uneasy. It had never happened before: he would come and he would speak, and he would go. But half an hour had passed. The sun had risen, everybody was feeling hot. There was silence superficially, but everybody was uncomfortable inside, chattering inside, asking, "Why is Buddha silent today?"

And he sat there under his tree with a flower in his hand and went on looking at the flower as if he was not even aware of those ten thousand disciples who had gathered to listen. They had come from very, very faraway villages. From all over the country, they had gathered.

Then somebody said, somebody gathered courage and said, "Why are you not speaking? We are waiting." Buddha is reported to have said, "I am speaking. This half hour, I have been speaking."

It was too paradoxical. It was patently absurd – he had remained silent, he had not said anything. But to say to Buddha, "You are talking absurdities," was not possible. The disciples again remained silent, more troubled now.

And suddenly one disciple, Mahakashyapa, started laughing. Buddha called him near, gave him the flower and said, "Whatsoever can be said, I have said to others, and that which cannot be said I have given to you." He only gave the flower, but this flower is just a symbol. With the flower he had given some significance also. This flower was just a sign, but he had conveyed something else which cannot be conveyed by words.

You also know certain feelings which cannot be conveyed. When you are deep in love, what do you do? You will feel it meaningless to simply go on saying, "I love you, I love you." And if you say it too much the other will get bored. And if you go on repeating the other will think you are just a parrot. And if you continue the other will think that you don't know what love is.

When you feel love it is meaningless to say that you love. You have to do something – something significant. It may be a kiss, it may be a hug, it may be just taking the other's hand into your hands, not doing anything, but it is a significance. You are conveying something which cannot be conveyed by words.

Buddha conveyed something which cannot be conveyed by

words. He gave the flower. It was a gift. That gift is visible; something invisible is passing with that gift.

When you take the hand of your friend in your hand, it is visible. Just taking the hand of your friend in your hand doesn't make much sense, but something else is passing. It is an exchange. Some energy, some feeling, something so deep that words cannot express it is passing. This is a sign, the hand is just a sign. Significance is invisible, it is passing. It is not a message, it is a gift, it is grace.

Buddha has given himself, he has not given any message. He has poured himself into Mahakashyapa. And Mahakashyapa became capable of receiving this for two reasons. One was that he remained totally silent while Buddha was silent. Others were also apparently silent, but they were not; they were continuously thinking, "Why is Buddha silent?" They were looking at each other, making gestures – "What has happened to Buddha? Has he gone mad? He has never been so silent."

Nobody was silent. Only Mahakashyapa, in that great assembly of ten thousand monks, was silent. He was not troubled, he was not thinking. Buddha was looking at the flower and Mahakashyapa was looking at Buddha. And you cannot find a greater flower than Buddha. That was the highest flowering of human consciousness. So Buddha went on looking at the flower and Mahakashyapa went on looking at Buddha. Only two persons were not thinking. Buddha was not thinking; he was looking. And Mahakashyapa was not thinking; he was also looking. This was the one thing that made him capable of receiving.

And the second thing was that he laughed. If silence cannot become celebration, if silence cannot become a laughter, if silence cannot become a dance, if silence cannot become an ecstasy, then it is pathological. Then it will become sadness. Then it will turn into a disease. Then silence will not be alive, it will be dead.

You can become silent just by becoming dead, but then you will not receive Buddha's grace. Then the divine cannot descend in you. The divine needs two things: silence and a dancing silence – a silence, alive. And he was both in that moment. He was silent, and when everybody was serious he laughed. Buddha poured *himself*: that is not a message.

Attain these two things then I can pour myself into you. Be silent, and don't make that silence a sad thing. Allow it to be laughing and dancing. The silence must be childlike, full of energy, vibrant, ecstatic. It should not be dead. Then, only then, can what Buddha did to Mahakashyapa be done to you.

My whole effort is that somebody, someday will become Mahakashyapa. But it is not a message.

The fourth question:

Osho,
You have often said that most scriptures have a lot of what are called "interpolations." Do the Yoga Sutras of Patanjali also suffer from this defect, and how will you deal with it?

No, Patanjali's Yoga Sutras are absolutely pure. No one has ever interpolated anything into them. There are reasons it cannot be done. First, Patanjali's Yoga Sutras is not a popular scripture. It is not a Gita, it is not a Ramayana, it is not a Bible. The common masses have never been interested in it. When the common masses are interested in something, they make it impure. It is bound to be so because then the scripture has to be dragged down to their level.

Patanjali's Yoga Sutras has remained only for experts; only a few chosen ones will get interested in it. Not everybody is going to be interested. And if by chance you happen to accidentally have Patanjali's Yoga Sutras, you can read only a few pages and then you will throw it away. It is not for you. It is not a story, it is not a drama, it is not an allegory. It is a simple, scientific treatise, only for the few. And the way it has been written is such that those who are not ready for it will turn their back automatically.

A similar case has happened in this century with Gurdjieff. For thirty years continuously he was preparing one book. A man of the caliber of Gurdjieff can do that work in three days. Even three days may be more than enough. Lao Tzu had done it: in three days the whole Tao Te Ching was written. Gurdjieff could have done it in three days; there was no difficulty – but for thirty years he was writing his first book. And what was he doing? He would write one chapter, and then he would allow it to be read before his disciples. The disciples would be listening to the chapter and he would be looking at the disciples. If they could understand, he would change it. That was the condition: if they could understand he would change it. If he saw that they were following it, then it was wrong. Continuously, for thirty years, every chapter was read a thousand and one times, and every time he was watching. When the book became completely impossible, that no one could read and understand it, then it was ready.

Even a very intelligent person will have to read it at least seven times; then glimpses of meaning will start coming. And that too will be just glimpses. If he wants to penetrate more, then he will have to practice whatsoever Gurdjieff has said, and through practice meanings will become clear. And it will take at least one's whole life to come to the total understanding of what he has written.

This type of book cannot be interpolated. Really, it is said that very few people have read his first book completely. It is difficult; it is one thousand pages. So when the first edition was published, he published it with a condition: only one hundred pages, the introductory part, was cut open. All other pages were not cut open, they were left uncut. Only one hundred pages were cut, and a note was given on the book, "If you can read the one hundred pages and still think to read ahead, then cut open the other pages. Otherwise, return the book to the publisher and take your money back."

It is said that there are very few people alive who have read the whole book completely. It is written in such a way that you will get fed up. Reading twenty, twenty-five pages, it is enough; and this man seems to be mad.

These are sutras, Patanjali's sutras; everything has been condensed in a seed. Somebody was asking me, "Patanjali has condensed sutras..." Just the other day somebody came and asked me, "...and you speak so much on those sutras." I have to, because he has made a tree a seed, and I have to make the seed again a tree.

Each sutra is condensed, totally condensed. You cannot do anything in it, and no one is interested to. Just to keep the book always pure, this was one of the methods. And for many thousands of years the book was not written, it was just memorized by disciples; it was given from one to the other just as a memory. It was not written, so nobody could do anything to it. It was a sacred memory, preserved. And even when the book was written it was written in such a way that if you put something in it, it will be found immediately.

Unless a person of the caliber of Patanjali tries that, it cannot be done. You cannot do it. Just think, if you have one Einstein formula, what can you do to it? If you do anything, it will be immediately caught. Unless a mind like Einstein tries to play with it nothing can be done. The formula is complete, nothing can be added, nothing can be deleted. In itself, it is a unit. Whatsoever you do, you will be caught.

These are seed formulas. If you add a single word, anyone who is working on the path of Yoga will immediately come to know that this is wrong.

I will tell you one anecdote...

It happened just in this century. One of the greatest poets of India, Rabindranath Tagore, translated his own book, *Gitanjali*, from Bengali to English. He translated it himself, and then he was a little hesitant whether the translation was okay or not. So he asked C. F. Andrews, one of the friends and disciples of Mahatma Gandhi, "Just go through it. How has the translation come out?" C. F. Andrews was not a poet, he was an Englishman, well educated, knowing the language, the grammar and everything, but he was not a poet.

So at four spots, on four points, he told Rabindranath to change certain words: "They are ungrammatical, and English people will not follow them." So Rabindranath simply changed whatsoever Andrews suggested. He changed four words in all in his translation. Then he went to London, and in a poets' gathering which had been arranged by one of the English poets of his time, Yeats, the translation was read for the first time.

When the whole translation was read, everybody listened and Rabindranath asked, "Have you any suggestions? Because this is just a translation and English is not my mother tongue."

And it is very difficult to translate poetry. Yeats, who was a poet of the same caliber as Rabindranath, said, "Only at four points is something wrong" – and those were exactly the four words that Andrews had suggested!

Rabindranath couldn't believe it. He said, "How, how could you find out? Because these are the four words I have not translated: Andrews suggested and I have put them in."

Yeats said, "The whole poetry is a flow, only these four are like stones; the flow is broken. It seems somebody else has done the work. Your language may not be grammatical, your language is not one hundred percent right – it cannot be, that we can understand – but it is one hundred percent poetry. These four words have come from a schoolmaster. The grammar has become right but the poetry has gone wrong."

With Patanjali, you cannot do anything. Anyone who is working on Yoga will find immediately that someone else who doesn't know anything has interpolated something. There are very few books which are still pure, and the purity has been retained. This is one of them. Nothing has been changed, not a single word, nothing has been added. It is as Patanjali meant it to be.

This is a work of objective art. When I say a work of objective art, I mean a certain thing. Every precaution has been taken. While these sutras were condensed, every precaution has been taken so that they could not be destroyed. They have been constructed in such a way that anything foreign, any foreign element will become a jarring note. But I say if a man like Patanjali tries, he can do that.

But a man like Patanjali will never try such a thing. Only lesser minds always try to interpolate. And lesser minds can try that, and the thing can continue, interpolated, only when it becomes a mass thing. The masses are not aware, cannot be aware. Only Yeats became aware that something was wrong in the poetry of Rabindranath. There were many others present in the gathering; no one else was aware.

This is a secret cult, a secret heritage. And the book is written, but the book form has not been thought to be reliable. There are still persons alive who have got Patanjali's sutras directly from their master, not from the book. And the tradition has yet remained alive, and it will continue because books are not reliable. Sometimes books can be lost. Many things can go wrong with books.

So there is a secret tradition, and that tradition has been maintained. And those who know through the words of their master, they go on continuously checking whether there is something wrong or something has been changed in the book form.

This has not been maintained for other scriptures. The Bible has so many interpolations that if Jesus comes back he will not be able to understand what has happened, how these things have come in, because not until three hundred years after Jesus died was the Bible recorded for the first time. In these three hundred years many things disappeared. Even his disciples have different stories to tell.

Buddha died. Two hundred years after his death his words were recorded. There are many schools, many scriptures, and no one can say which is true and which is false. But Buddha was talking to the masses, so he is not condensed like Patanjali. He was talking to the masses, to the ordinary, common people. He was elaborating things, in detail. In those details many things can be added, many things can be deleted, and no one will become aware that something has been done.

But Patanjali was not talking to the masses. He was talking to a very select few, a group, a group of very few persons, just like Gurdjieff. Gurdjieff never talked before the masses. A very selected group of his disciples was able to listen to him, and that too with many conditions. No meeting was ever declared beforehand. If he was going to talk this night, at eight-thirty, then nearabout eight o'clock you would get the indication that Gurdjieff was going to talk somewhere. And you have to reach there immediately because at eight-thirty the doors would be closed. And these thirty minutes were never enough. And when you reached you might find that he had canceled. Next day, again...

Once he continually cancelled for seven days. The first day four hundred people came, the last day only fourteen. By and by they got discouraged. And then it seemed impossible that he was going to talk. The last day, only fourteen people were there. When he looked, he said, "Now the right amount of people are left. You could wait for seven days and you were not discouraged, so now you have earned it. Now I will speak, and only these fourteen will be able to listen to this series. Now no one is to be informed that I have started speaking."

This type of work is different. Patanjali worked with a very closed circle. That's why no religion has come out of it, no organization. Patanjali has no sect. Such a tremendous force, but he remained closed within a small group. And he worked it out in such a way that the purity should be maintained. It has been maintained up to now.

The last question:

Osho,
Would you please explain the working of that unknown
force which keeps the human mind attracted, attached to
worldly things and habits, in spite of being fully aware

that the ultimate result is nothing but misery?

The awareness is not total, the awareness is just intellectual. Logically you follow, "Whatsoever I am doing is leading me to misery," but this is not your existential experience. Just rationally you understand. If you were reason alone then there would be no problem, but you are "unreason" also. If you had only a conscious mind then it would be okay; you have an unconscious mind also. The conscious mind knows that you are going into misery every day by your own efforts; you are creating your own hell. But the unconscious is not aware, and the unconscious is nine times more than your conscious mind. And that unconscious goes on persisting in its own habits.

You decide not to be angry again because anger is doing nothing but poisoning your own system. It gives you misery. But the next time someone insults you the unconscious will put aside your conscious reasoning, it will erupt, and you will be angry. That unconscious has not known about your decision at all, and that unconscious remains the active force.

The conscious mind is not active. It only thinks, it is a thinker; it is not a doer. So what has to be done? Just by thinking consciously that something is wrong you are not going to stop it. You will have to work at a discipline, and through discipline this conscious knowledge will penetrate like an arrow into the unconscious.

Through discipline, through Yoga, through practice, the conscious decision will reach into the unconscious, and when it reaches into the unconscious only then will it be of any use. Otherwise you will go on thinking one thing and you will go on doing something quite the contrary.

St. Augustine says, "Whatsoever good I know, I always think to do it – but whenever the opportunity to do it comes I always do whatsoever is wrong." This is the human dilemma.

And Yoga is the path to bridge the conscious with the unconscious. When we go deeper into the discipline you will become aware how this can be done. And this *can* be done. So don't rely on the conscious, it is inactive; the unconscious is the active. Change the unconscious, only then will your life have a different meaning. Otherwise you will be in more misery. Thinking something and doing something else will constantly create chaos, and by and by you will lose self-confidence. By and by you will feel that you are absolutely incapable, impotent, you cannot do anything. A self-condemnation will arise. You will feel guilty.

And guilt is the only sin.

Enough for today.

CHAPTER 7

an ecstasy is born

*Their cessation is brought about by persistent
inner effort and non-attachment*

*Of these two, abhyasa, the inner practice,
is the effort to be firmly established in oneself.*

*It becomes firmly grounded when continued for a long
time, without interruption and with reverent devotion.*

M an is not only his conscious mind. He has also nine times more than the conscious – the unconscious layer of the mind. Not only that, man has the body, the *soma,* in which this mind exists. The body is absolutely unconscious. Its working is almost non-voluntary. Only the surface of the body is voluntary; the inner sources are non-voluntary, you cannot do anything about them, your will is not effective.

This pattern of man's existence has to be understood before one can enter into oneself. And the understanding should not remain only intellectual. It must go deeper, it must penetrate the unconscious layers; it must reach to the very body itself.

Hence, the importance of *abhyasa*, constant inner practice. These two words are very significant: *abhyasa* and *vairagya*. *Abhyasa* means constant inner practice, and *vairagya* means non-attachment, desirelessness. The coming sutras of Patanjali are concerned with these two most significant concepts, but before we enter the sutras it has to be firmly grasped that this, the pattern of human personality, is not totally intellectual.

If it were only intellect then there would be no need for *abhyasa* – constant, repetitive effort. You can understand anything immediately if it is rational, through the mind, but just that understanding won't do. You can understand easily that anger is bad, poisonous, but this understanding is not enough for the anger to leave you, to disappear. In spite of your understanding the anger will continue, because the anger exists in many layers of your unconscious mind, and not only in the mind, but in your body also.

The body cannot understand just by verbal communication. Only your head can understand; the body remains unaffected. And unless understanding reaches to the very roots of the body you cannot be transformed. You will remain the same. Your ideas may go on changing but your personality will persist. And then a new conflict will arise and you will be in more turmoil than ever, because now you can see what is wrong and still you persist in doing it, you go on doing it. A self-guilt and condemnation is created. You start hating yourself, you start thinking yourself a sinner. And the more you understand, the more condemnation grows, because you see how difficult it is, almost impossible, to change yourself.

Yoga does not believe in intellectual understanding. It believes in bodily understanding, in a total understanding in which your wholeness is involved. Not only do you change in your head, but the deep sources of your being also change.

How can they change? Constant repetition of a particular practice becomes non-voluntary. If you do a particular practice constantly, just repeating it continuously, by and by it drops from the conscious, reaches to the unconscious and becomes part of it. Once it becomes part of the unconscious it starts functioning from that deep source.

Anything can become unconscious if you go on repeating it continuously. For example, your name has been repeated so constantly from your childhood that now it is not part of the conscious, it has become part of the unconscious. You may be sleeping with one hundred persons in a room, and if somebody comes and calls "Ram? Is Ram there?" ninety-nine persons who are not concerned with the name will go on sleeping. They will not be disturbed. But the person who has the name Ram will suddenly ask, "Who is calling me? Why are you disturbing my sleep?"

Even in sleep, he knows his name is Ram. How has this name reached so deep? – just by constant repetition. Everybody is repeating his name, everybody is calling it; and he himself, introducing himself – continuous use. Now it is not conscious, it has reached to the unconscious.

The language, your mother tongue, becomes a part of the unconscious. Whatsoever else you learn later on will never be so unconscious, it will remain conscious. That's why your unconscious language will continuously affect your conscious language. If a German speaks English it is different, if a Frenchman speaks English it is different, if an Indian speaks English it is different. The difference is not in English, the difference is in their innermost patterns. The Frenchman has a different pattern, unconscious pattern that affects it. So whatsoever you learn later on will be affected by your mother tongue. And if you fall unconscious, then only your mother tongue can penetrate.

I remember one of my friends who was a Maharashtrian. He was in Germany for twenty years, or even more. For twenty years he used the German language. He had completely forgotten his own mother tongue, Marathi. He couldn't read it, he couldn't talk it. Consciously, the language was completely forgotten because it was not used.

Then he became ill, and in that illness sometimes he would become unconscious. Whenever he would become unconscious, a totally different type of personality would evolve. He would start behaving in a different way. In his unconscious he would utter words from Marathi, not from German. When he was unconscious then he would utter words which are from the Marathi language. And after his unconsciousness, when he would come back to the conscious, for a few minutes he would not be able to understand German.

Constant repetition in childhood goes deeper, because the child really has no conscious. He has more of the unconscious just near the surface; everything enters into the unconscious. As he learns, as he gets educated, the conscious will become a thicker layer, and then there will be less and less penetration towards the unconscious.

Psychologists say that almost fifty percent of your learning is finished by your seventh year of age. By the seventh year of your life you have known almost half of the things that you are ever going to know. Half your education is finished, and this half is going to be the base. Now everything else will just be imposed on it and the deeper pattern of childhood will remain.

That's why modern psychology, modern psychoanalysis, psychiatry, all try to penetrate into your childhood, because if you are mentally ill, somewhere the seed is to be found in your childhood. The pattern must be located there in your childhood. Once that deep pattern is located, then something can be done and you can be transformed.

But how to penetrate it? Yoga has a method. That method is called *abhyasa*. *Abhyasa* means the constant, repetitive practice of a certain thing. Why, through repetition, does something become unconscious? There are a few reasons for it.

If you want to learn something you will have to repeat it. Why? If you read a poem just once, you may remember a few words here and there. But if you read it twice, thrice, many more times, then you can remember lines, paragraphs. If you repeat it a hundred times then you will remember it as a whole pattern. If you repeat it even more then it may continue, persist in your memory for years. You may not be able to forget it.

What is happening? When you repeat a certain thing, the more you repeat, the more it is engraved on the brain cells. A constant repetition is a constant hammering. Then it is ingrained, it becomes a part of your brain cells. And the more it becomes a part of your brain cells, the less consciousness is needed. Your consciousness can move; now it is not needed.

So whatsoever you learn deeply, you need not be conscious for it. In the beginning if you learn how to drive a car, then it is a conscious effort. That's why it is so much trouble, because you have to be alert continuously and there are so many things to be aware of – the road, the traffic, the mechanism, the wheel, the accelerator, the brakes and the rules and regulations of the road. You have to be constantly alert about everything. As you are so much involved in it, it becomes arduous, it becomes a deep effort.

But by and by you will be able to completely forget everything. You will drive, driving will become unconscious. You need not bring your mind to it – you can go on thinking anything you like, you can be anywhere you like and the car will move unconsciously. Now your body has learned it. Now the whole mechanism knows it. It has become an unconscious learning.

Whenever something becomes so deep that you need not be conscious about it, it falls into the unconscious. And once a thing has fallen into the unconscious it will start changing your being, your life, your character. And the change will be effortless now, you need not be concerned with it. You will simply move in the directions where the unconscious is leading you.

Yoga has worked very much on *abhyasa*, constant repetition. This constant repetition is just to bring your unconscious into work. And when the unconscious starts functioning you are at ease. No effort is needed, things become natural. It is said in old scriptures that a sage is not one who has a good character, because even that consciousness shows that the "anti" still exists, the opposite still exists. A sage is one who cannot do bad, cannot think about it. The goodness has become unconscious, it has become like breathing. Whatsoever he does will be good. It has become so deep in his being that no effort is needed, it has become his life. So you cannot say a sage is a good man. He doesn't know what is good, what is bad. Now there is no conflict. The good has penetrated so deeply that there is no need to be aware about it.

If you are aware about your goodness, the badness still exists side by side. There is a constant struggle. And every time you have to move into action you have to choose: "I have to do good, I have not to do bad." And this choice is going to be a deep turmoil, a struggle, a constant inner violence, inner war. And if there is conflict you cannot be at ease, at home.

Now we should enter the sutra. The cessation of mind is Yoga, but how can the mind cease?

> *Their cessation is brought about by persistent*
> *inner practice and non-attachment.*

Two things: how can the mind cease with all its modifications? – first, *abhyasa*, persistent inner practice, and second, non-attachment.

Non-attachment will create the situation, and persistent practice is the technique to be used in that situation. Understand both.

Whatsoever you do, you do because you have certain desires. And those desires can be fulfilled only by doing certain things. Unless those desires are dropped your activities cannot be dropped. You have some investment in those activities, in those actions. This is one of the dilemmas of human character and mind – that you may want to stop certain actions because they lead you into misery.

But why do you do them? You do them because you have certain desires, and those desires cannot be fulfilled without doing them. So there are two things. One, you have to do certain things. For example, anger. Why do you get angry? You get angry only when somewhere, somehow, someone creates a hindrance. You are going to achieve something and someone creates a hindrance. Your desire is obstructed; you get angry.

You can get angry even with things. If you are moving and you are trying to reach somewhere immediately and a chair comes in the way, you get angry with the chair. You try to unlock the door and the key is not working, you become angry with the door. It is absurd, because to be angry with a thing is nonsense. Anything that creates any type of obstruction creates anger.

You have a desire to reach, to do, to achieve something. Whosoever comes in between you and your desire appears to be your enemy, and you want to destroy him. This is what anger means: you want to destroy the obstacles. But anger leads to misery, anger becomes an illness so you want not to be angry.

But how can you drop anger if you have desires, goals? If you have desires and goals, then anger is bound to be there because life is complex; you are not alone here on this earth. Millions of people are striving for their own desires; they criss-cross each other, they come into each other's path. If you have desires then anger is bound to be there, frustration is bound to be there, violence is bound to be there. And your mind will think to destroy whosoever comes in your path.

This attitude to destroy the obstacle is anger. But anger creates misery, because you have been angry for millions of years. It has become a deep-rooted so you want not to be angry. But just wanting not to be angry will not be of much help, because anger is part of a greater pattern – of a mind which desires, a mind which has goals, a mind which wants to reach somewhere. You cannot drop anger.

So the first thing is not to desire. Then half of the possibility of anger is dropped; the base is dropped. But then too, it is not that anger will necessarily disappear because you have been angry for millions of years. It has become a deep-rooted habit. You may drop desires but anger will still persist. It will not be so forceful, but it will persist because now it is a habit. It has become an unconscious habit. For many, many lives you have been carrying it. It has become your heredity. It is in your cells, the body has taken it, and it is now chemical and physiological. Just by dropping your desires your body is not going to change its pattern. The pattern is very old; you will have to change this pattern also.

For that change, repetitive practice will be needed. Just to change the inner mechanism, repetitive practice will be needed – a reconditioning of the whole body-mind pattern. But this is possible only if you have dropped desiring.

Look at it from another point of view. One man came to me and he said, "I don't want to be sad, but I am always sad and depressed. Sometimes I cannot even feel why I am sad, but I am sad. No visible cause, nothing that I can pinpoint: "This is the reason." It seems that it has just become my style to be sad. I don't remember," he said, "that I was ever happy. And I don't want to be sad. It is a dead burden. I am the unhappiest person. So how I can drop it?"

So I asked him, "Have you got any investment in your sadness?"

He said, "Why should I have any investment?" But he had. I knew the person well. I had known the person for many years, but he was not aware that there was some vested interest in it. So he wants to drop sadness, but he is not aware why the sadness is there. He has been maintaining it for some other reasons which he cannot connect.

He needs love, but to be loved you need to be loving. If you ask for love you have to give love, and you have to give more than you can ask for. But he is a miser, he cannot give love. Giving is impossible to him; he cannot give anything. Just the word *giving*, and he will shrink within himself. He can only take, he cannot give. He is closed as far as giving is concerned.

But without love you cannot flower. Without love you cannot attain any joy, you cannot be happy. And he cannot love because love looks like giving something. It is a giving, a wholehearted giving of all that you have – your being also. He cannot give love, he cannot receive love. Then what to do? But he hankers, as everybody hankers, for love. It is a basic need, just like food. Without food your body will die, and without love your soul will shrink. It is a must.

He has created a substitute, and that substitute is sympathy. He cannot get love because he cannot give love, but he can get sympathy. Sympathy is a poor substitute for love. So he is sad: when he is sad people give him sympathy. Whosoever comes to him feels sympathetic because he is always crying and weeping. His mood is always that of a very miserable man. But he enjoys! Whenever you give him sympathy he enjoys it. He becomes more miserable, because the more he is miserable, the more he can get this sympathy.

So I told him, "You have a certain investment in your sadness. This whole pattern of sadness cannot be dropped, it is rooted somewhere else. Don't ask for sympathy. But you can stop asking for sympathy only when you start giving love, because it is a substitute. And once you start giving love, love will happen to you. Then you will be happy. Then a different pattern is created."

I have heard...

A man entered a car park. He was in a very ridiculous posture. It looked almost impossible to walk as he was walking, because he was crouching as if he was driving a car, his hands moving on some invisible wheel, his feet on some invisible accelerator, and he was walking. And it was so difficult, so impossible, how he was walking. A crowd gathered. He was doing something impossible and they asked the attendant, "What is the matter? What is this man doing?"

The attendant said, "Don't ask so loudly! This man loved cars in his past. He was one of the best drivers. He has even won a national prize in car racing. But now, due to some mental deficiency, he has been debarred. He is not allowed to drive a car, but the old hobby remains."

The crowd said, "If you know that then why don't you say to him, 'You don't have a car. What are you doing here?'"

The man said, "That's why I said don't speak so loudly! That I cannot do, because he gives me one rupee per day to wash the car. That I cannot do; I cannot say, 'You have no car.' He is going to park the car and then I will wash it."

That one-rupee investment is there. You have many investments in your misery also, in your anguish also, in your illness also. And then you go on saying, "We don't want – we don't want to be angry, we don't want to be this and that." But unless you come to know how all these things have happened to you, unless you see the whole pattern, nothing can be changed.

The deepest pattern of the mind is desire. You are whatsoever you are because you have certain desires, a group of desires. Patanjali says the first thing is non-attachment. Drop all desire, don't be attached and then, *abhyasa*.

For example, someone comes to me and he says, "I don't want to collect more fat on my body, but I go on eating. I want to stop it but I go on eating."

The wanting is superficial; there is a pattern inside, the reason he goes on eating more and more. And if he stops even for a few days, then again, with more gusto, he eats. And he will collect more weight than he has lost through a few days fasting or dieting. And this has been continuous, for years. It is not just a question of eating less. Why is he eating more? The body doesn't need it, then somewhere in the mind food has become a substitute for something. He may be afraid of death. People who are afraid of death eat more because eating seems to be the base of life. The more you eat, the more alive – this is the arithmetic in their mind – because if you don't eat you die. So not eating is equivalent to death and more eating is equivalent to more life. So if you are afraid of death you will eat more, or if nobody loves you, you will eat more.

Food can become a substitute for love because the child, in the beginning, comes to associate food and love. The first thing the child is going to be aware of is the mother, the food from the mother and the love from the mother. Love and food enter his consciousness simultaneously. And whenever the mother is loving she gives more milk. The breast is given happily. But whenever mother is angry, non-loving, she snatches the breast away.

Food is taken away whenever mother is not loving, food is given whenever she is loving: love and food become one. In the mind, in the child's mind, they become associated. So whenever the child gets more love he will reduce his food, because the love is so much that the food is not needed. Whenever love is not there he will eat more, because a balance has to be kept. If there is no love at all then he will fill his belly.

You may be surprised to know that whenever two persons are in love they lose fat. That's why girls start gathering fat the moment they are married. When love is settled, they start getting fat because now there is no need. Love and the world of love are, in a way, finished.

In the countries where divorce has become more prevalent, the women have better figures. In the countries where divorce is not prevalent, women don't bother at all about their figures because when divorce is possible then the women will have to find new lovers; they are figure conscious. The search for love helps the figure. When love is settled, it is finished in a way. You need not worry about the body, you need not take any care.

So this person may be afraid of death. Maybe he is not in any deep, intimate love with anyone. And these two are again connected: if you are in deep love you are not afraid of death. Love is so fulfilling that you don't care what is going to happen in the future. Love itself is the fulfillment. Even if death comes it can be welcomed. But if you are not in love then death creates a fear because you have not even loved yet and death is approaching near. Death will finish it, and there will be no time and no future after it.

If there is no love the fear of death will be more. If there is love there will be less fear of death. If there is total love, death disappears. These are all connected inside. Even very simple things are deeply rooted in greater patterns.

Mulla Nasruddin was standing before his veterinary doctor with his dog and insisting, "Cut off the tail of my dog!"

The doctor was saying, "But why, Nasruddin? If I cut off the tail of your dog, this beautiful dog will be destroyed. He will look ugly. And why are you insisting?"

Nasruddin said, "Between you and me – don't say this to anybody – I want the dog's tail to be cut off because my mother-in-law is going to come soon and I don't want any sign of welcome in my house. I have removed everything. Only this dog with his wagging tail can welcome my mother-in-law."

Even a dog's tail has a pattern of many relationships. If Nasruddin cannot welcome his mother-in-law even through his dog then he cannot be in love with his wife, it is impossible. If you are in love with your wife you will welcome the mother-in-law, you will be loving towards her.

Things that are simple on the surface are deeply rooted in complex things, and everything is interrelated. So just by changing a thought nothing is changed. Unless you go to the complex pattern, uncondition it, recondition it, create a new pattern, only then can a new life arise out of it. So these two things have to be done.

Non-attachment, non-attachment about everything – that doesn't mean that you stop enjoying. That misunderstanding has been there, and Yoga has been misinterpreted in many ways. One is this: it seems as if Yoga is saying that you die to life because non-attachment means then you don't desire anything. If you don't desire anything, if you are not attached to anything, if you don't love anything, then you will be just a dead corpse. No, that is not the meaning.

Non-attachment means don't be dependent on anything, and don't make your life and happiness dependent on anything. Preference is okay, attachment is not okay. When I say preference is okay I mean you can prefer – you *have* to prefer. If many people are there, you have to love someone, you have to choose someone, you have to be friendly with someone. Prefer someone, but don't get attached.

What is the difference? If you get attached then it becomes an obsession: if the person is not there you are unhappy. If you miss the person, you are in misery. And attachment is such a disease that if the person is not there you are in misery and if the person *is* there you are indifferent. Then it is okay, it is taken for granted. If the person is there it is okay, no more than that; if the person is not there then you are in misery – this is attachment.

Preference is just the reverse: if the person is not there you are okay, if the person is there you feel happy, thankful. If the person is there you don't take it for granted. You are happy, you enjoy it, you celebrate it. But if the person is not there, you are okay. You don't demand, you are not obsessed, you can also be alone and happy. You would have preferred that the person was there, but this is not an obsession.

Preference is good, attachment is disease. And a man who lives with preference lives life in deep happiness, you cannot make him miserable. You can only make him happy; you cannot make him miserable. A person who lives with attachment cannot be made happy, you can only make him more miserable. And you know this, you know this well. If your friend is there you don't enjoy him much, if the friend is not there you miss him.

A girl came to me a few days ago. She had seen me two months ago, with her boyfriend. And they were constantly fighting with each other, and the fight had become just an illness, so I told them to be separate for a few weeks. They said it was impossible to live together so I sent them away separately.

The girl was here on Christmas Eve and she said, "These two months, I have missed my boyfriend so much. I am thinking of him constantly. He has started to appear even in my dreams. This has never happened before. When we were together I never saw him in my dreams; in my dreams I was making love to other men. But now my boyfriend is constantly in my dreams. Now allow us to live together again."

So I told her, "It is okay with me, you can live together again. But just remember this: you were living together just two months ago and you were never happy."

Attachment is a disease. When you are together you are not happy. If you have riches you are not happy, you will be miserable if you are poor. If you are healthy you never feel thankfulness. If you are healthy you never feel grateful to existence, but if you are ill you are condemning the whole life and existence; everything is meaningless and there is no God.

Even an ordinary headache is enough to cancel all Gods. But when you are happy and healthy you never feel like going to a church or a temple, just to give thanks: "I am happy and I am healthy, and I have not earned these. These are simply gifts from you."

Mulla Nasruddin once fell in a river, and he was about to drown. He was not a religious man, but suddenly, at the verge of death, he cried loudly, "Allah, God, please save me, help me, and from today I will now pray and I will do whatsoever is written in the scripture."

While he was saying this "God help me," he caught hold of a branch overhanging the river. And when he grabbed and came towards safety he felt relaxed, and he said, "Now it is okay. Now you need not worry."

Again he said to God, "Now you need not worry. Now I am safe."

Suddenly the branch broke and he fell again. So he said, "Can't you take a simple joke?"

But this is how our minds are moving.

Attachment will make you more and more miserable; preference will make you more and more happy. Patanjali is against attachment, not against preference. Everybody has to prefer. You may like one food, you may not like another, but this is just a preference. If the food of your liking is not available then you will take your second choice. And you will be happy because you know the first was not available, and whatsoever is available had to be enjoyed. You will not cry and weep. You will accept life as it happens to you.

But a person who is constantly attached with everything never enjoys anything and always misses. The whole life becomes a continuous misery. If you are not attached you are free, you have much energy, you are not dependent on anything. You are independent, and this energy can be moved into inner effort. It can become a practice; it can become *abhyasa*. What is *abhyasa*? *Abhyasa* is fighting the old habitual pattern. Every religion has developed many practices, but the base is this sutra of Patanjali.

For example, whenever you get angry, make it a constant practice that before entering into anger you will take five deep breaths. A simple practice, apparently not related to anger at all. And somebody can even laugh: "How is it going to help?" But it *is* going to help. Whenever you feel anger arising, before you express it take five deep exhalations and inhalations.

What will it do? It will do many things. Anger can be there only if you are unconscious – and this is a conscious effort. Just before anger arises, consciously breathe in and out five times: this will make your mind alert, and with alertness anger cannot enter. This will not only make your mind alert, it will also make your body alert, because the more oxygen there is in the body, the more alert the body becomes. In this alert moment suddenly you will feel that the anger has disappeared.

Secondly, your mind can only be one-pointed. Mind cannot think of two things simultaneously, it is impossible for the mind. It can change from one to another very swiftly but it cannot have two points together in the mind simultaneously. One thing at a time – mind has a very narrow window, only one thing at a time. So if anger is there, anger is there. If you breathe in and out five times suddenly the mind is with the breathing. It has diverted, now it is moving in a different direction. And even if you again move to anger, you cannot be the same again because the moment has been lost.

Gurdjieff says, "When my father was dying he told me to remember only one thing: 'Whenever you are angry, wait for twenty-four hours and then do whatsoever you like. Even if you want to murder, go and murder – but wait for twenty-four hours.'"

Twenty-four hours is too long; twenty-four seconds will do. Just the waiting changes you. The energy that was flowing towards anger has taken a new route. It is the same energy – it can become anger, it can become compassion. Just give it a chance.

So the old scriptures say, "If a good thought comes to your mind don't postpone it, do it immediately. And if a bad thought comes to your mind postpone it, never do it immediately." But we think we are very cunning or very clever – whenever a good thought comes we postpone it.

Mark Twain has written in his memoirs that he was listening to a priest in a church for ten minutes. The lecture was just wonderful and he thought in his mind, "Today I am going to donate ten dollars. This priest is wonderful. This church must be helped!" He decided he was going to donate ten dollars after the lecture. Ten minutes more and he started thinking that ten dollars would be too much, five would do. Ten minutes more and he thought, "This man is not even worth five dollars."

Now he was not listening, now he was worried about those ten dollars. He had not told anybody, but now he was convincing himself that this was too much. He says, "By the time the lecture finished, I decided not to give anything. And when the man came before me to take the donations, the man who was moving around, I even thought to take a few dollars and escape from the church!"

Mind is continuously changing. It is never static, it is a flow. If something bad is there, wait a little. You cannot fix the mind, mind is a flow. You just wait! Just wait a little and you will not be able to do wrong. If some good is there and you want to do it, do it immediately, because mind is changing and after a few minutes you will not be able to do it. So if it is a loving and kind act, don't postpone it. If it is something violent or destructive, postpone it a little.

If anger comes, postpone it even for five breaths and you will not be able to act on it. This will become a practice. Every time anger comes first breathe five times in and out then you are free to act. Go on continuously and it becomes a habit, you need not even think: the moment anger enters, immediately your mechanism will start breathing fast, deep. Within years it will become absolutely impossible for you to be angry. You will not be able to be angry.

Any practice, any conscious effort, can change your old patterns. And this is not a work which can be done immediately, it will take time. Because you have created your pattern of habits in many, many lives, if even in one life you can change it, it is too soon.

My sannyasins come to me and they say, "When will it happen?" and I say, "Soon." And they say, "What do you mean by your 'soon'? – because for years you have been telling us 'soon.'"

If even in one life it happens, it is soon. Whenever it happens it has happened before its time, because you have created this pattern in so many lives. They have to be destroyed and recreated. So any amount of time – even lives – is not too late.

Their cessation is brought about by persistent
inner practice and non-attachment.

Of these two, abhyasa, the inner practice,
is the effort to be firmly established in oneself.

The essence of *abhyasa* is to be centered in oneself. Whatsoever happens, you should not move immediately. First you should be centered in yourself, and from that centering you should look around and then decide.

Someone insults you and you are pulled by his insult. You have moved without consulting your center. You have moved without even for a single moment going back to the center, and then moving.

Abhyasa means inner practice. Conscious effort means, "Before I move out, I must move within. First, movement must be toward my center. First, I must be in contact with my center. Centered there, I will look at the situation and then decide." And this is such a tremendous, transforming phenomenon. Once you are centered within everything appears different, the perspective is changed: it may not look like an insult, the man may just look stupid. Or if you are really centered, you will come to know that he is right:

"This is not an insult. He has not said anything wrong."

I have heard – I don't know whether it is true or not, but I have heard this anecdote:

One newspaper was continuously writing against Richard Nixon, continuously defaming him, condemning him. So Richard Nixon went to the editor and said, "What are you doing? You are telling lies about me and you know it well!"

The editor said, "Yes, we know that we are telling lies about you. But if we start telling truths about you, you will be in more trouble!"

So if someone is saying something about you he may be lying, but just look again: if he were really true, it might be worse. Or, whatsoever he is saying may apply to you. But when you are centered, you can also look dispassionately about yourself.

Patanjali says that of these two, *abhyasa*, the inner practice, is the effort to become firmly established in oneself. Before moving into an act, any sort of act, move within yourself. First be established there, even if for only a single moment, and your action will be totally different. It cannot be the same unconscious pattern of old. It will be something new, it will be an alive response. Just try it. Whenever you feel that you are going to act or to do something first move within – because whatsoever you have been doing up until now has become robot-like, mechanical. You go on doing it continuously, in a repetitive circle.

For thirty days just note down in a diary, from the morning to the evening, for thirty days, and you will be able to see the pattern. You are moving like a machine, you are not a man. Your responses are dead. Whatsoever you do is predictable. And if you study your diary penetratingly, you may be able to decipher the pattern: that Monday, every Monday, you are angry, every Sunday you feel sexual, every Saturday you are fighting. Or in the morning you are good, in the afternoon you feel bitter, by the evening you are against the whole world – you may see the pattern. Once you see the pattern then you can just observe that you are working like a robot. And being a robot is what misery is. You have to be conscious, not a mechanical thing.

Gurdjieff used to say, "As he is, man is a machine." You become man only when you become conscious. And this constant effort to be established in oneself will make you conscious, will make you non-mechanical, will make you unpredictable, will make you free. Then someone can insult you and you can still laugh; you have never laughed before. Someone can insult you and you can feel love for the man; you have not felt that before. Someone can insult you and you can be thankful towards him. Something new is being born; now you are creating a conscious being within yourself.

But the first thing to do before moving into an act is to first be established, because to act means moving outward, moving without, moving toward others, going away from the self. Every act is a going away from the self. Before you go away have a look, have a contact, have a dip into your inner being. First be established.

Before every movement, let there be a moment of meditation: this is what *abhyasa* is. Whatsoever you do, before doing it close your eyes, remain silent, move within. Just become dispassionate, non-attached, so you can look as an observer, unprejudiced, as if you are not involved, you are just a witness. And then move!

One day, just in the morning, Mulla Nasruddin's wife said to Mulla, "In the night, while you were asleep, you were insulting me. You were saying things against me, swearing against me. What do you mean? You will have to explain."

Mulla Nasruddin said, "But who says that I was asleep? I was not asleep. Just that the things I want to say, I cannot say in the day. I cannot gather so much courage."

In your dreams, in your waking, you are constantly doing things, and those things are not done consciously. It is as if you are being forced to do them. Even in your dreams you are not free. This constant mechanical behavior is the bondage. So how to be established in oneself? – through *abhyasa*.

Sufis use it continuously whatsoever they say or do; they sit, they stand, whatsoever they do. Before a Sufi disciple stands he will take Allah's name, first he will take God's name. He will sit, he will take God's name. An action is to be done – even sitting is an action – sitting he will say, "Allah," standing, he will say, "Allah." If it is not possible to say it loudly he will say it inside. Every action is done through remembrance, and by and by, this remembrance becomes a constant barrier between him and the action. A division is created, a gap.

And the more this gap grows, the more he can look at his own action as if he is not the doer. With continuous repetition of "Allah," by and by he starts seeing that only Allah is the doer: "I am not the doer. I am just a vehicle or an instrument." And the moment this gap grows, all that is evil falls away. You cannot do evil. You can do evil only when there is no gap between the actor and the action. Then the good flows automatically.

The greater the gap between the actor and the action, the more good happens. Life becomes a sacred thing. Your body becomes a temple. Anything that makes you alert, established within yourself, is *abhyasa.*

> *Of these two, abhyasa, the inner practice,*
> *is the effort to be firmly established in oneself.*

> *It becomes firmly grounded when continued for a long*
> *time, without interruption and with reverent devotion.*

...when continued for a long time... How long? It will depend. It will depend on you, on each person, how long. The length of time will depend on the intensity. If the intensity is total then it can happen very soon, even immediately. If the intensity is not so deep then it will take a longer period.

I have heard...

A Sufi mystic, Junnaid, was taking a walk outside his village one morning. A man came running and asked Junnaid, "The capital of this kingdom is where? I want to reach the capital. How long will I still have to travel? How much time will it take?"

Junnaid looked at the man and, without answering him, again started walking. And the man was also going in the same direction, so the man followed. The man thought, "This old man seems to be deaf," so a second time he asked more loudly, "I want to know how much time it will take for me to reach the capital!"

But Junnaid still continued walking. After walking two miles with that man, Junnaid said, "You will have to walk at least ten hours."

The man said, "But you could have said that before."

Junnaid said, "How can I say it? First I must know your speed. It depends on your speed. So for these two miles I was watching what your speed is. Only now can I answer."

It depends on your intensity, your speed.

There are two things to be remembered. The first thing is: ...*when continued for a long time, without interruption*... This has to be remembered. If you interrupt, if you do it for some days and then leave it for some days, the whole effort is lost. And when you start again it is again a beginning.

If you are meditating and then you say, "For a few days there is no problem..." You feel lazy, you feel like sleeping in the morning and you say, "I can postpone, I can do it tomorrow." Even one day missed, you have undone the work of many days. Because you are not doing meditation today but you will be doing many other things, and those many other things belong to your old pattern, so a layer is created. Your yesterday and your tomorrow are cut off. Today has become a layer, a different layer. The continuity is lost, and when you start again tomorrow it is again a beginning. I see many persons starting, stopping, again starting. The work that can be done within months then takes years.

So this is to be remembered: ...*without interruption*... Whatsoever practice you choose, then choose it for your whole life, and just go on hammering on it, don't listen to the mind. Mind will try to persuade you, and mind is a great seducer. It can give all kinds of reasons: that today it is a must not to do it because you are feeling ill, there is headache, you couldn't sleep in the night, you have been so very tired so you can just rest today. These are tricks of the mind.

Mind wants to follow its old pattern. Why does the mind want to follow its old pattern? – because there is least resistance, it is easier. And everybody wants to follow the easier path, the easier course. It is easy for the mind just to follow the old, the new is difficult.

So mind resists everything that is new. If you are in practice, in *abhyasa*, don't listen to the mind, just go on doing. By and by this new practice will go deep in the mind, and mind will stop resisting it because then it will become easier. Then for mind it will be an easy flow. Unless it becomes an easy flow, don't interrupt. You can undo a long effort by a little laziness, so it must be uninterrupted.

And the second thing to be remembered: ...*with reverent devotion.*

You can do a practice mechanically, with no love, no devotion, no feeling of holiness about it, then it will take very long. Through love things penetrate easily in you. Through devotion you are open, more open, seeds fall deeper.

With no devotion you can do the same thing. For instance, in a temple you can have a hired priest. He will say prayers continuously for years with no result, with no fulfillment through it. He is doing as it is prescribed, but it is a work with no devotion. He may show devotion, but he is just a servant. He is interested in his salary, not in the prayer, not in the *puja,* not in the ritual. It is to be done, it is a duty, it is not a love. So he will do it for years. Even for his whole life he will be just a hired priest, a salaried man. In the end he will die as if he has never prayed. He may die in the temple, praying, but he will die as if he has never prayed because there was no devotion.

So don't do *abhyasa,* a practice, without devotion, because then you are unnecessarily wasting energy. Much can come out of it if devotion is there. What is the difference? The difference is between duty and love. Duty is something you have to do, you don't enjoy doing it. You have to carry it on somehow, you have to finish it soon. It is just an outward work. If this is the attitude then how can it penetrate in you?

A love is not a duty – you enjoy it. There is no limit to its enjoyment, there is no hurry to finish it. The longer it lasts, the better. It is never enough; you always feel something more, something more can be done. It is always unfinished. If this is the attitude then things go deep in you. The seeds reach to the deeper soil. Devotion means you are in love with a particular *abhyasa,* a particular practice.

I observe that with many of the people I work with this division is very clear. Those who practice meditation as if they are doing just a technique can do it for years with no change happening. It may help a little, bodily. They may be healthier, their physiques will get some benefits out of it, but it is just an exercise. And then they come to me and they say, "Nothing is happening."

Nothing will happen, because the way they are doing it is something outside, just like work – as if they go to the office at eleven and leave the office at five. They can go to the meditation hall with no involvement. They can meditate for one hour and come back, with no involvement. It is not in their heart.

The other category is of those people who do it with love. It is not a question of doing something. It is not quantitative, it is qualitative: how much you are involved, how deeply you love it, how much you enjoy it – not the goal, not the end, not the result, but the very practice.

Sufis say, "Repetition of the name of God, repetition of the name of Allah, is in itself the bliss." They go on repeating and they enjoy. This becomes their whole life, just the repetition of the name.

Nanak says, "*Nam smaran*" – remembering the name is enough. You are eating, you are going to sleep, you are taking your bath, and continuously your heart is filled with the remembrance. Just go on repeating "Ram" or "Allah" or whatsoever, not as a word, but as a devotion, as a love. Your whole being feels filled, vibrates with it, it becomes your deeper breath. You cannot live without it. And by and by it creates an inner harmony, a music. Your whole being starts falling into harmony; an ecstasy is born.

You are filled with a humming sensation, a sweetness surrounds you, and by and by this sweetness becomes your nature. Then whatsoever you say, it becomes the name of Allah. Whatsoever you say, it becomes the remembrance of the divine.

Any practice ...*without interruption and with reverent devotion*, is very difficult for the Western mind. They can understand practice, they cannot understand "reverent devotion." They have completely forgotten that language, and without that language practice is just dead. Western seekers come to me and they say, "Whatsoever you say we will do," and they follow it exactly as it is said. But they work on it just as if they were working on any other know-how, a technique. They are not in love with it, they have not become mad, they are not lost in it. They remain manipulating.

They are the master and they go on manipulating the technique just as they would manipulate any mechanical device. Just as you can push a button and the fan starts – there is no need for any reverent devotion for the button or for the fan. And you do everything in life like that, but *abhyasa* cannot be done that way. You have to be so deeply related with your *abhyasa*, your practice, that you become secondary and the practice becomes primary, that you become the shadow and the practice becomes the soul – as if it is not you who is doing the practice, but the practice is going on by itself and you are just a part of it, vibrating with it. Then it may be that no time is needed.

With deep devotion, results can follow immediately. In a single moment of devotion you can undo many lives of the past. In a deep moment of devotion you can become completely free from the past.

But it is difficult to explain that reverent devotion. There is friendship, there is love – and there is a different quality of friendship plus love which is called reverent devotion. Friendship and love exist between equals. Love is between opposite sexes, friendship is with the same sex but on the same level; you are equals.

Compassion is just the opposite of reverent devotion. Compassion exists from a higher source towards a lower source. Compassion is like a river flowing from the Himalayas to the ocean. A buddha is compassion. Whosoever comes to him, his compassion is flowing downwards. Reverence is just the opposite – as if the Ganges is flowing from the ocean towards the Himalayas, from the lower to the higher.

Love is between equals, compassion is from the higher to the lower, devotion is from the lower to the higher. Compassion and devotion have both disappeared and only friendship remains. And without compassion and devotion, friendship is just hanging in between, dead, because the two poles are missing. And it can exist, living, only between those two poles.

If you are in devotion then sooner or later compassion will start flowing towards you. If you are in devotion then some higher peak will start flowing towards you. But if you are not in devotion compassion cannot flow towards you, you are not open to it.

All *abhyasa*, all practice, is to become the lowest so the highest can flow in you. Become the lowest. As Jesus says, "Only those who stand last will become the first in my kingdom of God."

Become the lowest, the last. Suddenly, when you are the lowest, you are capable of receiving the highest. And only to the lowest depth is the highest attracted, pulled. It becomes the magnet.

"With devotion" means you are the lowest. That is why Buddhists choose to be beggars. Sufis have chosen to be beggars – just the lowest, the beggars – and we have seen that in those beggars the highest has happened. But this is their choice. They have put themselves in the last. They are the last ones, not in competition with anybody, just valley-like, low, lowest.

That's why in the old Sufi sayings it is said, "Become a slave of God" – just a slave, repeating his name, constantly thanking him, constantly feeling gratitude, constantly filled with so many blessings that he has poured upon you.

And with this reverence, devotion; uninterrupted *abhyasa*, practice: Patanjali says these two, *vairagya* and *abhyasa*, help the mind to cease. And when mind ceases, for the first time you are really that which you are meant to be, that which is your destiny.

Enough for today.

CHAPTER 8

stop, and it is here!

The first question:

Osho,
Patanjali has stressed the importance of non-attachment,
that is, cessation of desire, for being rooted in oneself.
But is non-attachment really at the beginning of the
journey or at the very end?

The beginning and the end are not two things. The beginning is the end, so don't divide them and don't think in terms of duality. If you want to be silent in the end, you will have to begin with silence from the very beginning. In the beginning the silence will be like a seed, in the end it will become a tree. But the tree is hidden in the seed, so the beginning is just the seed.

Whatsoever the ultimate goal, it must be hidden here and now, just in you, in the very beginning. If it is not there in the beginning you cannot achieve it in the end. Of course there will be a difference: in the beginning it can only be a seed, in the end it will be the total flowering. You may not be able to recognize it when it is a seed, but it is there whether you recognize it or not. So when Patanjali says non-attachment is needed in the very beginning of the journey, he is not saying that it will not be needed in the end.

Non-attachment in the beginning will be with effort, non-attachment in the end will be spontaneous. In the beginning you will have to be conscious about it, in the end there will be no need to be conscious about it. It will be just your natural flow.

In the beginning you have to practice it. Constant alertness will be needed. There will be a struggle with your past, with your patterns of attachment; there will be fight. In the end there will be no fight, no alternative, no choice. You will simply flow in the direction of desirelessness. That will have become your nature.

But remember, whatsoever is the goal has to be practiced from the very beginning. The first step is also the last, so one has to be very careful about the first step. If the first is in the right direction, only then will the last be achieved. If you miss the first step you have missed all.

This will come again and again to your mind, so understand it deeply because Patanjali will say many things which look like ends. Nonviolence is the end, when a person becomes so compassionate, so deeply love-filled that there is no violence, no possibility of violence. Love or nonviolence is the end, but Patanjali will say to practice it from the very beginning.

The goal has to be in your view from the very beginning. The first step of the journey must be absolutely devoted to the goal, directed to the goal, moving towards the goal. It cannot be the absolute thing in the beginning, neither does Patanjali expect it. You cannot be totally non-attached, but you can try. The very effort will help you.

You will fall many times, you will again and again get attached. And your mind is such that you may even get attached with non-attachment. Your pattern is so unconscious, but effort, conscious effort, will by and by make you alert and aware. And once you start feeling the misery of attachment then there will be less need for the effort, because no one wants to be miserable, no one wants to be unhappy.

We are unhappy because we don't know what we are doing, but the longing in every human being is for happiness. No one longs for misery; everybody creates misery because we don't know what we are doing. Or we may be moving in desires towards happiness, but the pattern of our mind is such that we actually move towards misery.

From the very beginning, when a child is born, is brought up, wrong mechanisms are fed into his mind, wrong attitudes are fed in. No one is trying to make him wrong, but wrong people are all around. They cannot be anything else, they are helpless.

A child is born without any pattern. There is just a deep longing for happiness but he doesn't know how to achieve it; the how is unknown. This much is certain: he knows that happiness is to be attained. He will struggle his whole life but he doesn't know the means, the methods of how it is to be achieved, where it is to be achieved, where he should go to find it. The society teaches him how to achieve happiness, and the society is wrong.

A child wants happiness, but we don't know how to teach him to be happy. And whatsoever we teach him becomes the path towards misery. For example, we teach him to be good. We teach him not to do certain things and to do certain things, without ever thinking, "Is it natural or unnatural?" We say, "Do this, don't do that." Our "good" may be unnatural – and if whatsoever we teach as good is unnatural, then we are creating a pattern of misery.

For example, a child is angry and we say, "Anger is bad, don't be angry." But anger is natural, and just by saying "Don't be angry" we are not destroying anger, we are just teaching the child to suppress it. Suppression will become misery because whatsoever is suppressed becomes poisonous. It moves into the very chemicals of the body, it is toxic. And by continuously teaching "Don't be angry" we are teaching him to poison his own system.

One thing we are not teaching him is how not to be angry. We are simply teaching him how to suppress the anger. And we can force him because he is dependent on us. He is helpless; he has to follow us. If we say, "Don't be angry," then he will smile, but that smile will be false. Inside he is bubbling, inside he is in turmoil, inside there is fire and he is smiling outside.

We are making a hypocrite out of a small child. He is becoming false and divided. He knows that his smile is false. His anger is real but the real has to be suppressed and the unreal has to be forced. He will be split. And by and by the split will become so deep, the gap will become so deep, that whenever he smiles he will smile a false smile.

And if he cannot be really angry then he cannot be really anything, because reality is condemned. He cannot express his love, he cannot express his ecstasy: he has become afraid of the real. If you condemn one part of the real the whole reality is condemned, because reality cannot be divided and a child cannot divide.

One thing is certain: the child has come to understand that he is not accepted. As he is, he is not acceptable. The real is somehow bad, so he has to be false. He has to use faces, masks. Once he has learned this the whole life will move in a false dimension. And the false can only lead to misery; the false cannot lead to happiness. Only the true, authentically real, can lead you towards ecstasy, towards the peak experiences of life: love, joy and meditation, whatsoever you name them.

Everybody is brought up in this pattern, so you long for happiness but whatever you do creates misery. The first step towards happiness is to accept oneself. The society never teaches you to accept yourself. It teaches you to condemn yourself, to be guilty about yourself, to cut out many parts of yourself. It cripples you, and a crippled man cannot reach to the goal. And we are all crippled.

Attachment is misery. But from the very beginning attachment is demanded of the child. The mother says to the child, "Love me, I am your mother." The father says, "Love me, I am your father," as if someone automatically becomes lovable if he is a father or she is a mother.

Just being a biological mother doesn't mean much or just being a biological father doesn't mean much. To be a father is to pass through a great discipline: one has to be lovable. To be a mother is not just to reproduce: to be a mother means a great training, a great inner discipline, one has to be lovable.

If the mother is lovable then the child will love without any attachment. And wherever he will find that someone is lovable, he will love. But mothers are not lovable, fathers are not lovable; they have never thought in those terms – that love is a quality.

You have to create it, you have to become it. You have to grow. Only then can you create love in others. It cannot be demanded. If you demand it, it can become an attachment, but not love.

So the child will love the mother because she is his mother. The mother or the father becomes the goals. These are relationships, not love. Then he becomes attached to the family, and the family is a destructive force because the family of the neighbor is separate; it is not lovable because you don't belong to it. Then your community, your nation...but the neighboring nation is the enemy.

You cannot love the whole humanity: your family is the root cause. And the family has not been bringing you up to be a lovable person and a loving person, it is forcing some relationships. Attachment is a relationship, and love is a state of mind. Your father will not say to you, "Be loving," because if you are loving you can be loving to anybody. Even sometimes the neighbor may be more lovable than your father, but the father cannot accept this, that anybody can be more lovable than him, because *he* is your father. So relationship has to be taught, not love.

This is *my* country, that's why I have to love this country. If simply love is taught, then I can love any country. But the politician will be against it because if I love any country, if I love this earth, then I cannot be dragged into war. So the politicians will teach, "Love this country. This is *your* country, you are born here. You belong to this country, your life, your death, belongs to this country" – so he can sacrifice you for it.

The whole society is teaching you relationships, attachments, not love. Love is dangerous because it knows no boundaries. It can move, it is freedom. So your wife will tell you, "Love me because I am your wife." The husband is telling the wife, "Love me because I am your husband." Nobody is teaching love.

If simply love is taught, then the wife can say, "But the other person is more lovable." If the world were really free to love, then just being a husband could carry *any* meaning, and just being a wife wouldn't mean anything. Then love would freely flow. But that is dangerous – society cannot allow it, the family cannot allow it, the religions cannot allow it. So in the name of love they teach attachment, and then everybody is in misery.

When Patanjali says non-attachment, he is not anti-love. *Really*, he is for love. Non-attachment means be natural, loving, flowing, but don't get obsessed and addicted. Addiction is the problem. Then it is like a disease. You cannot love anybody except your child – this is addiction. Then you will be in misery. Your child can die, then there is no possibility for your love to flow. Even if your child is not going to die, he will grow. And the more he grows the more he will become independent. And then there will be pain. Every mother suffers, every father suffers.

The child will become an adult, he will fall in love with some woman. And then the mother suffers, a competitor has entered. But this is because of attachment. If a mother really loves the child she will help him to be independent. She will help him to move in the world and to make as many love contacts as possible, because the more you love the more you are fulfilled. And when her child falls in love with a woman she will be happy, she will dance with joy.

Love never gives you misery, because if you love someone you love his happiness. If you are attached to someone you don't love his happiness, you love only your selfishness; you are concerned only with your own egocentric demands.

Freud discovered many things. One of them is mother or father-fixation. He says the most dangerous mother is the one who forces the child to love her so much that he becomes fixated and he will not be able to love anybody else. So there are millions of people suffering because of such fixations.

As far as I have been trying to study many people, I have found that almost all the husbands, at least ninety-nine percent, are trying to find their mothers in their wives. Of course, you cannot find your mother in your wife; your wife is not your mother. But a deep fixation with the mother, and then they are dissatisfied with the wife because she is not mothering them. And every wife is searching for the father in the husband, and no husband is your father. And if she is not satisfied with the fathering then she is dissatisfied.

These are fixations. In Patanjali's language, he calls them attachments. Freud calls them fixations. The words differ but the meaning is the same. Don't get fixed, be flowing. Non-attachment means you are not fixed. Don't be like ice cubes, be like water, flowing. Don't be frozen.

Every attachment becomes a frozen thing, dead. It is not vibrating with life, it is not a constantly moving response. It is not alive moment to moment, it is fixed. You love a person: if it is love then you cannot predict what is going to happen the next moment. It is impossible to predict, moods change like weather. You cannot say the next moment also that your lover will be loving to you. He may not feel like loving the next moment, you cannot expect it.

If he also loves you the next moment it is good, you are thankful. If he is not loving in the next moment nothing can be done, you are helpless. You have to accept the fact that he is not in the mood. Nothing to cry about, simply there is no mood for love! You accept the situation. You don't force the lover to pretend, because pretension is dangerous.

If I feel loving towards you I say, "I love you," but the next moment I can say, "No, I don't feel any love in this moment." So there are only two possibilities: either you accept my non-loving mood, or you force: whether you love me or not, at least show that you love me." If you force me then I become false and the relationship becomes a pretension, a hypocrisy. Then we are not true to each other. And how can two persons who are not true to each other be in love? Their relationship will have become a fixation.

Wife and husband are fixed, dead, everything is certain. They are behaving towards each other as if they are things. When you come to your home, your furniture will be the same as when you left because furniture is dead. Your house will be the same because the house is dead. But you cannot expect your wife to be the same, she is alive, a person. And if you expect her to be the same as she was when you left the house then you are forcing her to be just furniture, just a thing. Attachment forces the related persons to be things and love helps the persons to be freer, to be more independent, to be truer. But truth can only be in constant flow, it can never be frozen.

When Patanjali says non-attachment he is not saying to kill your love. Rather, on the contrary, he is saying, "Kill all that poisons your love, kill all the obstacles, destroy all the obstacles that kill your love." Only a yogi can be loving; the worldly person cannot be loving, he can only be attached.

Remember this: attachment means fixation and you cannot accept anything new in it, only the past. You don't allow the present; you don't allow the future to change anything. And life is change, only death is unchanging.

If you are unattached, then moment to moment you move without any fixation. Every moment life will bring new happinesses, new miseries. There will be dark nights and there will be sunny days, but you are open, you don't have a fixed mind. When you don't have a fixed mind even a miserable situation cannot give you misery because you don't have anything to compare with it. You were not expecting something against it so you cannot be frustrated.

You get frustrated because of your demands. You think that when you come home, your wife will be just standing outside to welcome you. And if she is not standing there outside to welcome you,

you cannot accept it. This gives you frustration and misery. You demand, and through demand you create misery. And demand is possible only if you are attached. You cannot demand with persons who are strangers to you. Only with attachment does demand come in; that is why all attachments become hellish.

Patanjali says be non-attached. That means be flowing, accepting whatsoever life brings. Don't demand and don't force. Life is not going to follow you; you cannot force life to be according to you. It is better to flow with the river rather than pushing it. Just flow with it, and much happiness becomes possible. There is already much happiness all around you, but you cannot see it because of your wrong fixations.

But in the beginning this non-attachment will only be a seed; in the end non-attachment becomes desirelessness. In the beginning non-attachment means non-fixation, in the end non-attachment will mean desirelessness, no desire. In the beginning no demand, in the end no desire.

But if you want to reach to this end of no-desire, start from no-demand. Try Patanjali's formula even for twenty-four hours, just for twenty-four hours, flowing with life, not demanding anything. Whatsoever life gives, feeling grateful, thankful. Just moving for twenty-four hours in a prayerful state of mind, not asking, not demanding, not expecting, and you will have a new opening. Those twenty-four hours will become a new window. And you will feel how ecstatic you can become.

But you will have to be alert in the beginning. It cannot be expected that non-attachment, for the seeker, can be a spontaneous act.

The second question:

> Osho,
> How is it that an enlightened one gives of himself to one
> only, as Lord Buddha did in the case of Mahakashyapa?
> Really, this Buddhist tradition of one disciple receiving
> the light continued for eight generations. Was it not
> possible for a group to be its recipient?

No, it is never possible, because the group has no soul, the group has no self. Only the individual can be the recipient, the receiver, because only the individual has the heart. A group is not a person.

You are here, I am talking, but I am not talking to the group because with the group there can be no communication. I am talking to each individual here. You have gathered in a group but you are not hearing me as a group, you are hearing me as individuals. Really, the group doesn't exist, only individuals exist. Group is just a word; it has no reality, no substance. It is just the name of a collectivity.

You cannot love a group, you cannot love a nation, you cannot love humanity. But there are persons who claim that they love humanity. They deceive themselves because there is no one like humanity anywhere, there are only human beings. Go and search: you will never find humanity somewhere. Really, the persons who claim that they love humanity are the persons who cannot love a person. They are incapable of being in love with a person. So they use big names – humanity, nation, universe. They may even love God but they cannot love a person, because to love a person is arduous, difficult; it is a struggle.

You have to change yourself. To love humanity presents no problem. There is no humanity, you are alone. Truth, beauty, love or anything that is significant always belongs to the individual, only individuals can be recipients.

Ten thousand monks were there when Buddha poured his being into Mahakashyapa, but the group was incapable. No group can be capable, because consciousness is individual, awareness is individual. Mahakashyapa rose to the peak where he could receive Buddha. Other individuals can also rise to that peak, but no group.

Religion basically remains individualistic, and it cannot be otherwise. That is one of the basic fights between Communism and religion. Communism thinks in terms of groups, societies, collectivities, and religion thinks in terms of the individual person, the self. Communism thinks that the society can be changed as a whole, and religion thinks only individuals can be changed. Society cannot be changed as a whole because society has no soul, it cannot be transformed. In fact there is no society, only individuals.

Communism says there are no individuals, only society. Communism and religion are absolutely antagonistic, and this is the antagonism. If Communism becomes prevalent, then individual freedom disappears. Then only the society exists. The individual is not allowed really to be there. He can exist only as a part, as a cog in the wheel. He cannot be allowed to be a self.

I have heard...

A man reported in a Moscow police station that his parrot was missing, so he was directed to the clerk concerned. The clerk wrote, and he asked, "Does the parrot speak also? He talks?"

The man became afraid, a little troubled, uncomfortable. He said, "Yes, he talks. But whatsoever political opinion he expresses, those political opinions are strictly his own."

A parrot! This individual was afraid because what a parrot speaks means those political opinions must belong to his master. A parrot simply imitates. No individuality is allowed in Communism, you cannot have your opinions. Opinions are the concern of the state, the group mind, and the group mind is the lowest thing possible. Individuals can reach to the peaks. No group has ever become Buddha-like or Jesus-like; only an individual peaks.

Buddha is giving his whole life's experience to Mahakashyapa because there is no other way. It cannot be given to any group; it cannot be, it is just impossible. Communication, communion can only be between two individuals. It is a personal, deeply personal faith. The group is impersonal. And remember that a group can do many things: madness is possible with the group, but buddhahood is not possible. A group can be mad but a group cannot be enlightened.

The lower the phenomenon the more the group can participate in it. All great sins are committed by the group, not by individuals. An individual can murder a few people, but an individual cannot become "fascism," he cannot murder millions. Fascism can murder millions, and with good conscience!

After the Second World War all the war criminals proclaimed that they were not responsible, that they were just following orders from above. They were just part of the group. Even Hitler and Mussolini were very sensitive in their private lives. Hitler used to listen to music, he loved music. He even used to paint sometimes, he loved painting. Seems impossible, Hitler loving painting and music; so sensitive, and killing millions of Jews without any inconvenience, without any discomfort in his conscience, not even a prick. He was "not responsible." Then he was just the leader of a group.

When you are moving in a crowd you can commit anything because you feel, "The crowd is doing it. I am just part of it." Alone you would think thrice whether to do it or not. In the crowd responsibility is lost, your individual thinking is lost, your discrimination is lost, your awareness is lost. You have become just a part of a crowd. Crowds can go mad. Every country knows, every period knows crowds can go mad, and then they can do anything, but it has never been heard that crowds can become enlightened.

The higher states of consciousness can be achieved only by individuals. More responsibility has to be felt, more individual responsibility, more conscience. The more you feel you are responsible, the more you feel you have to be aware, the more you become individual.

Buddha communicates his silent experience with Mahakashyapa, his silent *sambodhi,* his silent enlightenment, because Mahakashyapa has also become a peak, a height, and two heights could now meet. And this will always be so. So if you want to reach higher peaks don't think in terms of groups, think in terms of your own individuality. A group can be helpful in the beginning, but the more you grow the less and less a group can be helpful.

A point comes when the group cannot be of any help, you are left alone. And when you are totally alone and you start growing in your loneliness, for the first time you are crystallized. You have become a soul, a self.

The third question:

Osho,
Practice is a sort of conditioning at the physical and
mental levels, and it is through conditioning that society
makes man its slave. In that case, how can Patanjali's
practice be an instrument of liberation?

Society conditions you to make a slave out of you, an obedient member, so the question seems valid: how can a continuous reconditioning of the mind make you liberated? The question seems valid only because you are confusing two types of conditioning.

You have come to me, you have traveled a path. When you go back you will travel the same path again. The mind can ask, "The path which brought you here, how can the same path take you back?" The path will be the same; your direction will be different, quite the opposite. While you were coming towards me you were facing towards me, when going back you will be facing the opposite direction, but the path will be the same.

The society conditions you to make you an obedient member, to make you a slave; it is just a path. The same path has to be traveled to make you free, only the direction will be the opposite. The same method has to be used to "uncondition" you.

I remember one parable...

Once Buddha went to his monks, he was going to deliver a sermon. He sat under his tree. He had a handkerchief in his hand. He looked at the handkerchief, the whole congregation also looked at what he was doing. Then he tied five knots in the handkerchief and then he asked two questions: one, "Is the handkerchief the same as when there were no knots in it or is it different?"

One *bhikkhu,* one monk, said, "In a sense it is the same because the quality of the handkerchief has not changed. Even with knots it remains the same, the same handkerchief. The inherent nature remains the same. But in a sense it has changed because something new has appeared: knots were not there, now knots are there. So superficially it has changed but deep down it has remained the same."

Buddha said, "This is the situation of the human mind: deep down it remains unknotted but the quality remains the same."

When you become a buddha, an enlightened one, you will not have a different consciousness. The quality will be the same. The difference is only that now you are a knotted handkerchief, your consciousness has a few knots.

A second thing Buddha asked: "What should I do to unknot this handkerchief?"

Another monk said, "Unless we know what you have done to knot it we cannot say anything, because the reverse process will have to be applied. The way you have knotted it has to be known first, because that will again be the way, in the reverse order, to unknot it."

So Buddha said, "This is the second thing. How you have come into this bondage has to be understood. How you are conditioned in your bondage has to be understood, because the same will be the process, in reverse order, to uncondition you."

If attachment is the conditioning factor, then non-attachment will become the unconditioning factor. If expectation leads you into misery, then non-expectation will lead you out of your misery. If anger creates a hell within you, then compassion will create a heaven. So whatsoever the process of misery, the reverse will be the process of happiness. Unconditioning means you have to understand the whole knotted phenomenon of human consciousness as it is. This whole process of Yoga will be nothing but understanding the complex knots and then unknotting them, unconditioning them. It is not a reconditioning, remember. It is simply unconditioning; it is negative. If it is a reconditioning then you will become a slave again, a new type of slave in a new imprisonment. So this difference has to be remembered: it is unconditioning, not reconditioning.

Because of this, many problems have arisen. Krishnamurti says that if you do anything it will become a reconditioning, so don't do anything. If you do anything it will become a reconditioning: you may be a better slave but you will remain a slave. Listening to him many people have stopped all efforts, but that doesn't make them liberated. They are not liberated, the conditioning is there. They are not reconditioning. Listening to Krishnamurti, they have stopped, they are not reconditioning, but they are also not unconditioning. They remain slaves.

So I am not for reconditioning, neither is Patanjali for reconditioning. I am for unconditioning, and Patanjali is also for unconditioning. Just understand the mind, whatsoever its disease. Understand the disease, diagnose it, and move in the reverse order.

What is the difference? Take some actual example. You feel anger: anger is a conditioning, you have learned it. Psychologists say that it is a learning, it is a programmed thing. Your society teaches it to you. There are societies even now which never get angry, the members never get angry. There are societies, small tribal clans still in existence, which have never known any fight, have never fought a war.

In the Philippines, a small aboriginal tribe exists. For three thousand years it has not known any fight, not a single murder, not a single suicide. What has happened to it? They are the most peace-loving people and the happiest possible. From the very beginning their society never conditions them for anger. In that tribe, if even in your dream you kill someone, you have to go and ask his forgiveness – even in a dream! If you are angry with someone and fighting, the

next day you have to declare to the village that you have done something wrong. Then the village will gather together, and the wise men of
the village will diagnose your dream and they will suggest what is to
be done now. Even small children!

I was reading their dream analyses. They seem to be one of the
most penetrating people. A small child dreams, and in a dream he
sees the boy of the neighbor looking very sad. So he tells the dream
to his father in the morning: "I have seen the boy of the neighbor
looking very sad."

So the father thinks over it, closes his eyes, meditates, and then
he says, "If you have seen him sad, that means somehow his sadness is related to you. No one else has dreamed about him that he is
sad, so either knowingly or unknowingly you have done something
which creates his sadness. Or, if you have not done, in the future you
are going to do. So the dream is just a prediction for the future. Go
with many sweets, gifts. Give sweets and gifts to the boy and ask for
his forgiveness for something done in the past or for something
which you are going to do in the future."

So the boy goes, gives the fruits, sweets, gifts, and asks his forgiveness because somehow, in the dream, he is responsible for his
sadness. From the very beginning the children are brought up in this
way. If this tribe has existed without strife, fight, murder, suicide,
there is no wonder. They cannot conceive of it. A different type of
mind is functioning there.

Psychologists say that hate and anger are not natural. Love is
natural: hate and anger are just created. They are hindrances in love,
and society conditions you for them. Unconditioning means whatsoever the society has done it has done; there is no use to go on condemning it, it is already the case. And by simply saying that the
society is responsible, you are not helped. It has been done. Now,
right now, what can you do? – you can uncondition. So whatsoever
your problems, look deep in the problem, penetrate it, analyze it, and
see how you are conditioned for it.

For example, there are societies which never feel competitive.
Even in India there are aboriginal tribes where no competition exists.
Of course they cannot be very progressive in our measurement,
because our progress can only be through competition. They are not
competitive. Because they are not competitive they are not angry,
they are not jealous, they are not so hate-filled, they are not so

violent. They don't expect much, and whatsoever their life gives to them they feel happy and grateful.

But no matter what life gives to you, you will never feel grateful. You will always be frustrated because you can always ask for more. And there is no end to your expectations and desires. So if you feel miserable look into the misery and analyze it. What are the conditioning factors which are creating the misery? And it is not very difficult to understand it. If you can create misery, if you are so capable of creating misery, there is no difficulty in understanding it. If you can create it you can understand it.

Patanjali's whole standpoint is this: looking into the misery of man, it is found that man himself is responsible. He is doing something to create it. That doing has become habitual, so he goes on doing it. It has become repetitive, mechanical, robotic. If you become alert you can drop out of it. You can simply say, "I will not cooperate." The mechanism will start working.

Someone insults you: just stand still, remain silent – the mechanism will start, it will bring the past pattern. The anger will be coming, the smoke will arise and you will feel just on the verge of getting mad. But stand still. Don't cooperate and just look at what the mechanism is doing. You will feel wheels within wheels within you, but they are impotent because you are not cooperating.

Or if you feel it is impossible to remain in such a still state, then close your door, move into the room, have a pillow before you and beat the pillow, be angry with the pillow. And when you are beating, getting angry and mad with the pillow, just go on watching what you are doing, what is happening, how the pattern is repeating itself.

If you can stand still, that's the best. If you feel it is difficult, that you are pulled, then move into a room and be angry on the pillow. Because with the pillow your madness will be totally visible to you, it will become transparent. And the pillow is not going to react: you can watch more easily and there is no danger, no safety problem. You can watch: slowly, the rising of the anger and the decline of the anger.

Watch both, the rhythm. When your anger is exhausted and you don't feel like beating the pillow anymore, or you have started laughing or you feel ridiculous, then close your eyes, sit on the floor, and meditate on what has happened. Do you still feel anger for the person who has insulted you, or it is thrown onto the pillow? You will feel a certain calmness falling on you. And you will not feel angry now with the person concerned. Rather, you may even feel compassion for him.

One young American boy was here two years ago. He had escaped from America because of only one problem, one obsession: he was continuously thinking of murdering his father. The father must have been a dangerous man, must have suppressed this boy too much. In his dreams he was thinking of murdering his father, in his daydreams also he was thinking of murdering him. He escaped from his home just to separate from the father. Otherwise, any day, something could happen. The madness was there, it could erupt any moment.

He was here with me and I told him, "Don't suppress it." I gave him a pillow and said, "This is your father. Now do whatsoever you like." At first he started laughing, laughing in a mad way. And he said, "It looks ridiculous." I told him, "Let it be ridiculous. But it is in the mind, let it come out." For fifteen days continuously he was beating and tearing the pillow. And doing it, on the sixteenth day he came with a knife. I had not told him to, so I asked him, "Why this knife?"

He said, "Now don't stop me. Let me kill. Now the pillow is not a pillow for me. The pillow has actually become my father." That day he killed his father. And then he started crying, tears came to his eyes. He became calmed down, relaxed, and he told me, "I am feeling much love for my father, much compassion. Now allow me to go back."

He is back there now. The relationship has totally changed. What has happened? – just a mechanical obsession has been released.

If you can stand still when some old pattern grips your mind, it is good. If you cannot, then allow it to happen in a dramatic way, but alone, not with someone. Because whenever you enact your pattern, allow your pattern with someone, it creates new reactions and it is a vicious circle.

The most significant point is to be watchful of the pattern. Whether you are standing silently or acting out your anger and hate, be watchful, looking at how it uncoils. And if you can see the mechanism you can undo it.

All these steps in Yoga are just for undoing something which you have been doing. They are negative, nothing new is to be created. Only the wrong is to be destroyed, the right is already there. Nothing positive is to be done, only something negative. The positive is hidden there. It is just like a stream is there, hidden under a rock. You are not to create the stream. It is already there, knocking; it wants to be released and to become free and flowing. Just a rock is there, and this rock has to be removed. Once the rock is removed the stream starts flowing.

Bliss, happiness, joy, or whatsoever you call it, is already there flowing in you. Only some rocks are there: those rocks are the conditionings of the society. Uncondition them. If you feel attachment is the rock then make efforts for non-attachment. If you feel anger is the rock then make efforts for non-anger. If you feel greed is the rock then make efforts for non-greed. Just do the opposite. Don't suppress greed, just do the opposite, do something which is non-greed. Don't just suppress anger, do something which is non-anger.

In Japan, when someone gets angry, they have a traditional teaching. If someone gets angry, immediately he has to do something which is non-anger. And the same energy which was going to move into anger moves into non-anger. Energy is neutral. If you feel angry with someone and you want to slap his face, give him a flower and see what happens.

You wanted to slap his face, you wanted to do something: that was anger. Give him a flower and just watch what is happening within you; you are doing something which is of non-anger. And the same energy which was going to move your hand will move your hand; and the same energy which was going to hit him is now going to give the flower but the quality has changed. You have done something, and the energy has become neutral; if you don't do something then you suppress, and suppression is poisonous. Do something, but just the opposite. And this is not a new conditioning; it is just to uncondition the old. When the old has disappeared, the knots have disappeared, you need not worry for anything to do. Then you can flow spontaneously.

The last question:

Osho,
You said that the spiritual endeavor may take twenty to thirty years, or even lives, and even then it is early. But the Western mind seems to be result-oriented, impatient and too practical. It wants instantaneous results.

Religious techniques come and go like other fads in the
West. Then how do you intend to introduce Yoga to the
Western mind?

I am not interested in the Western mind or the Eastern mind: these
are just two aspects of one mind. I am interested in the mind. And this
Eastern–Western dichotomy is not very meaningful, not even significant now. There are Eastern minds in the West and there are Western
minds in the East. And now the whole thing has become a mess. The
East is now also in a hurry. The old East has disappeared completely.
I am reminded of one Taoist anecdote...

Three Taoists were meditating in a cave. One year passed. They
were silent, sitting, meditating. One day a horseman passed nearby.
They looked. One of the three hermits said, "The horse he was
riding was white." The other two remained silent.

After one year again, the second hermit said, "The horse was
black, not white."

Then one more year passed again. The third hermit said, "If there
are going to be discussions, I am leaving. If there is going to be some
bickering, I am leaving. I am leaving! You are disturbing my silence."

What did it matter whether the horse was white or black? Three
years! But this was the flow in the East. Time was not. The East was
not conscious of time at all. The East lived in eternity, as if time
was not passing. Everything was static.

But that East no longer exists; the West has corrupted everything.
The East has disappeared; through Western education everybody is
now Western. There are only a few people, like in the islands, who are
"Eastern" – they can be in the West, they can be in the East. Now they
are not in any way confined to the East. But the world as a whole, the
earth as a whole, has become Western.

Yoga says – and let it penetrate you very deeply because it will be
very meaningful – Yoga says the more impatient you are, the more
time will be needed for your transformation. The more in a hurry, the
more you will be delayed. Hurry itself creates such confusion that
delay will result. The less in a hurry, the earlier will be the results. If
you are infinitely patient, this very moment transformation can
happen. If you are ready to wait forever, you may not wait even for

this next moment. This very moment the thing can happen because it is not a question of time, it is a question of the quality of your mind.

Infinite patience, simply not hankering for the result gives you much depth. Hurry makes you shallow. You are in such a hurry that you cannot be deep. This moment, you are not interested here in this moment but in what is going to happen in the next. You are interested in the result. You are moving ahead of yourself; your movement is mad. So you may run too much, you may travel too much – you will not reach anywhere because the goal to be reached is just here. You have to drop into it, not to reach anywhere. And the dropping is possible only if you are totally patient.

I will tell you one Zen anecdote...

A Zen monk is passing through a forest. Suddenly he becomes aware that a tiger is following him, so he starts running. But his running is also of a Zen type, he is not in a hurry. He is not mad; his running also is smooth, harmonious. He is enjoying it. And it is said that the monk thought in the mind, "If the tiger is enjoying it, then why not I?"

And the tiger was following him. Then he came near a precipice. Just to escape the tiger he hung from the branch of a tree. And then he looked down and saw that a lion was standing there in the valley, waiting for him. Now the tiger had arrived; he was standing just near the tree on the hilltop. The monk was hanging in between, just holding a branch, and the lion was waiting for him deep down in the valley.

He laughed. Then he looked – two mice were just eating that branch, one white, one black. Then he laughed very loudly. He said, "This is life. Day and night, white and black mice cutting. And wherever I go death is waiting. This is life!" And it is said that he achieved a *satori*, the first glimpse of enlightenment.

This is life! Nothing to worry about, this is how things are. Wherever you go death is waiting, and even if you don't go anywhere day and night are cutting your life. So he laughs loudly.

Then he looks around, because now it is fixed. Now there is no worry. When death is certain, what is the worry? Only in uncertainty is there worry. If everything is certain there is no worry, now it has become destiny. So he looks for how to enjoy these few moments. He becomes aware of some strawberries just by the side of the branch, so he picks a few strawberries and eats them. They are the best of his life! He enjoys them, and it is said that he becomes enlightened in that moment.

He has become a buddha, because death is so near and even then he is not in any hurry. He can enjoy a strawberry. It is sweet, the taste of it is sweet. He thanks God. It is said in that moment that everything disappeared – the tiger, the lion, the branch, he himself. He had become the cosmos.

This is patience, absolute patience. Wherever you are, in that moment, enjoy not asking for the future. No futuring in the mind, just the present moment, the nowness of the moment, and you are satisfied. Then there is no need to go anywhere. Wherever you are, from that very point you will drop into the ocean, you will become one with the cosmos.

But the mind is not interested in here and now. The mind is interested somewhere in the future, in some results. So the question is, in a way, relevant for such a mind – it will be better to call it the modern mind rather than Western – the modern mind which is constantly obsessed with the future, with the result, not with the here and now.

How can this mind be taught Yoga? This mind can be taught Yoga because this future orientation is leading nowhere. And this future orientation is creating constant misery for the modern mind. We have created a hell, and we have created too much of it. Now either man will have to disappear from this planet Earth, or he will have to transform himself. Either humanity will have to die completely because this hell cannot be continued anymore, or we will have to go through a mutation.

Hence, Yoga can become very meaningful and significant for the modern mind because Yoga can save. It can teach you again how to be here and now, how to forget past and how to forget future and how to remain in the present moment with such intensity that this moment becomes timeless. The very moment becomes eternity.

Patanjali can become more and more significant. As this century comes to its closure, techniques about human transformation will become more and more important. They are already becoming, all over the world – whether you call them Yoga or Zen, or you call them Sufi methods or you call them Tantra methods. In many, many ways, all the old traditional teachings are erupting. Some deep need is there, and those who are thinking – anywhere, in any part of the world – have become interested in again finding out how humanity existed in the past with such beautitude, such bliss. With such poor conditions, how have such rich men existed in the past? And we, with such a rich situation, why are we so poor?

This is a paradox, the modern paradox: for the first time on the earth we have created rich, scientific societies, and yet they are the most ugly and most unhappy. And in the past there was no scientific technology, no affluence, nothing of comfort, but humanity was existing in such a deep, peaceful milieu, happy, thankful. What has happened? We could be happier than anyone, but we have lost contact with existence.

That existence is here and now, and an impatient mind cannot be in contact with it. Impatience is like a feverish, mad state of mind. You go on running, and even if the goal comes, you cannot stand there because the running has become just a habit. Even if you reach the goal you will miss it, you will pass it, because you cannot stop. If you can stop, the goal is not to be sought, it is there.

Zen master Hui-Hai has said, "Seek and you will lose, don't seek and you can get it immediately. Stop, and it is here. Run, and it is nowhere."

Enough for today.

this very life, the ultimate joy

*The first state of vairagya, desirelessness: cessation
from self-indulgence in the thirst for sensuous
pleasures, with conscious effort.*

*The last state of vairagya, desirelessness: cessation
of all desiring by knowing the innermost nature of
purush, the supreme self.*

*A*bhyasa and *vairagya* – constant inner practice and desirelessness: these are the two foundation stones of Patanjali's
Yoga. Constant inner effort is needed not because something
has to be achieved but because of wrong habits. The fight is not
against nature, the fight is against habits. Nature is there, every
moment available to flow in, to become one with it, but you have a
wrong pattern of habits. Those habits create barriers. The fight is
against these habits, and unless they are destroyed, the nature, your
inherent nature, cannot flow, cannot move, cannot reach to the destiny for which it is meant.

So remember the first thing: the struggle is not against nature.
The struggle is against wrong nurture, wrong habits. You are not

fighting yourself, you are fighting something else which has become fixed with you. If this is not understood rightly, then your whole effort can go in a wrong direction. You may start fighting with yourself, and once you start fighting with yourself you are fighting a losing battle. You can never be victorious. Who will be victorious and who will be defeated? You are both, the one who is fighting and the one with whom you are fighting. If both my hands start fighting, who is going to win?

Once you start fighting with yourself you are lost, and so many people, in their endeavors, in their seeking for spiritual truth, fall into that error. They become victims of this error, and start fighting with themselves. If you fight with yourself you will go more and more insane. You will be more and more divided, split, you will become schizophrenic. This is what is happening in the West.

Christianity – not Christ, Christianity – has taught to fight with oneself, to condemn oneself, to deny oneself. Christianity has created a great division between the lower and the higher; there is nothing lower and nothing higher in you. Christianity talks about the lower self and the higher self, or the body and the soul. But somehow Christianity divides you and then creates a fight. This fight is going to be endless, it will not lead you anywhere. The ultimate result can only be self-destruction, a schizophrenic chaos. That's what is happening in the West.

Yoga never divides you, but still there is a fight. The fight is not against your nature. On the contrary, the fight is for your nature. You have accumulated many habits; those habits are your achievement of many lives' wrong patterns. And because of those wrong patterns your nature cannot move spontaneously, cannot flow spontaneously, cannot reach to its destiny. These habits have to be destroyed. And these are only habits – they may look like nature to you because you are so addicted to them. You may have become identified with them, but they are not you.

This distinction has to be clearly maintained in the mind, otherwise you can misinterpret Patanjali. Whatsoever has come into you from without and is wrong has to be destroyed so that which is within you can flow, can flower. *Abhyasa*, constant inner practice, is against habits.

The second thing, the second foundation stone, is *vairagya*, desirelessness. That too can lead you in a wrong direction. And, remember, these are not rules, these are simple directions. When I say these are not rules I mean they are not to be followed like an obsession, their meaning and significance has to be understood, and that significance has to be carried in one's life. It is going to be different for everyone so it is not a fixed rule. You are not to follow it dogmatically. You have to understand its significance and then allow it to grow within you. The flowering is going to be different with each individual. So these are not dead, dogmatic rules, these are simple directions. They indicate the direction, they don't give you the detail.

I remember, once Mulla Nasruddin was working as a doorkeeper in a museum. The first day he was appointed he asked for the rules: "What rules have to be followed?" So he was given the book of rules that were to be followed by the doorkeeper. He memorized them, he took every care not to forget a single detail.

And the first day when he was on duty, the first visitor came. He told the visitor to leave his umbrella there outside with him at the door. The visitor was amazed. He said, "But I don't have any umbrella."

So Nasruddin said, "In that case, you will have to go back. Bring an umbrella because this is the rule. Unless a visitor leaves his umbrella here outside, he cannot be allowed in."

And there are many people who are rule-obsessed. They follow blindly. Patanjali is not interested in giving you rules. Whatsoever he is going to say are simply directions, not to be followed but to be understood. And out of that understanding, following will come. The reverse cannot happen: if you follow the rules, understanding will not come. If you understand the rules, the following will come; will come automatically, as a shadow.

Desirelessness is a direction. If you follow it as a rule then you will start killing your desires. Many have done that, millions have done that – they start killing their desires. Of course this is mathematical, this is logical. If desirelessness is to be achieved then the best way is to kill all desires. Then you will be without desires but you will also be dead. You have followed the rule exactly, but if you kill all desires you are killing yourself, you are committing suicide because desires are not only desires, they are the flow of life energy. Desirelessness is to be achieved without killing anything.

Desirelessness is to be achieved with more life, with more energy, not less.

For example, you can kill sex easily if you starve the body, because sex and food are deeply related. Food is needed for your survival, for the survival of the individual, and sex is needed for the survival of the race, of the species. They are both food, in a way. Without food the individual cannot survive and without sex the race cannot survive, but the primary is the individual. If the individual cannot survive then there is no question of the race.

So if you starve your body, if you give so little food to your body that the energy created by it is exhausted in day-to-day routine work, walking, sitting, sleeping; if no extra energy accumulates, then sex will disappear. Sex can be there only when the individual is gathering extra energy, more than he needs for his survival. Then the body can think of the survival of the race.

If you are in danger then the body simply forgets about sex; hence so much attraction for fasting, because if you fast sex disappears. But this is not desirelessness, this is just becoming more and more dead, less and less alive. In India, Jaina monks have been fasting continuously just for this end, because if you fast continuously and you are constantly on a starvation diet, sex disappears. Nothing else is needed, no transformation of the mind, no transformation of the inner energy, simply starving helps. Then you become habituated to starvation. And if you continuously do it for years, you will simply forget that sex exists. No energy is created, no energy moves to the sex center. There is no energy to move! The person exists just as a dead being. There is no sex.

But this is not what Patanjali means. This is not a desireless state. It is simply an impotent state, energy is not there. If you give food to the body, even though you may have starved the body for thirty or forty years, once you give the right food to the body, sex reappears immediately. You are not changed, the sex is just hidden there waiting for energy to flow. Whenever energy flows it will become alive again.

So what is the criterion? The criterion has to be remembered: be more alive, be more filled with energy, vital, and become desireless. Only then, if your desirelessness makes you more alive have you followed the right direction. If it simply makes you a dead person you have followed the rule. It is easy to follow the rule because no intelligence is required. It is easy to follow the rule because simple tricks can do it. Fasting is a simple trick. Nothing much is implied in it, no wisdom is going to come out of it.

There was an experiment in Oxford. For thirty days a group of twenty students, young healthy boys, were totally starved. After the seventh or eighth day they started losing interest in girls. Nude pictures were given to them and they were indifferent. And this indifference was not just bodily, even their minds were not interested.

There are now methods to judge the mind. Whenever a young boy, a healthy boy, looks at a nude picture of a girl, the pupils of his eyes become big. They are more open to receive the nude figure. And you cannot control your pupils, they are not voluntary. So you may say that you are not interested in sex, but a nude picture will show whether you are interested or not. And you cannot do anything voluntarily; you cannot control the pupils of your eyes. They expand, because something so interesting has come before them that they open more, the shutters open more to take more in. Now, women are not interested in nude men, they are interested in small babies, so if a beautiful baby's picture is given to them their eyes expand.

In the Oxford experiment, every precaution was taken to see whether the boys were interested, and there was no interest. By and by the interest declined more. Even in their dreams they stopped seeing girls, sexual dreams. By the second week, the fourteenth or fifteenth day, they were simply dead corpses. Even if a beautiful girl came nearby they would not look. If someone said a dirty joke they would not laugh. For thirty days they were starved, and on the thirtieth day the whole group was sexless. There was no sex in their minds, in their bodies.

Then food was given to them again: on the very first day they again became as they were. The next day they were interested, and the third day all that starving for thirty days had disappeared. Now not only were they interested, they were obsessively interested, as if this gap had helped. For a few weeks they were obsessively sexual, only thinking of girls and nothing else. When the food was in the body, girls became important again.

But this has been done in many countries all over the world. Many religions have followed this fasting. And then people start thinking that they have gone beyond sex. You can go beyond sex, but fasting is not the way. That's a trick. And this can be done in every way. If you are on a fast you will be less angry, and if fasting becomes habitual then many things from your life will simply drop because the base has dropped: food is the base.

When you have more energy you move in more dimensions. When you are filled with overflowing energy, your overflowing energy leads you into many, many desires. Desires are nothing but outlets for energy. Two ways are possible: one is that your desire changes and the energy remains, or energy is removed and the desire remains. Energy can be removed very easily. You can simply be operated on, castrated, and then sex disappears. Some hormones can be removed from your body. And that's what fasting is doing – some hormones disappear, then you can become sexless.

But this is not the goal of Patanjali. Patanjali says that energy should remain and desire disappears. Only when desire disappears and you are filled with energy can you achieve that blissful state that Yoga aims at. A dead person cannot reach to the divine. The divine can be attained only through overflowing energy, abundant energy, an ocean of energy.

So this is the second thing to remember continuously: don't destroy energy, destroy desire. It will be difficult. It is going to be hard, arduous, because it needs a total transformation of your being. But Patanjali is for it. So he divides his *vairagya*, his desirelessness, into two steps. We will enter the sutra.

The first sutra:

> *The first state of vairagya – desirelessness: cessation*
> *from self-indulgence in the thirst for sensuous*
> *pleasures, with conscious effort.*

Many things are implied and have to be understood. One: the indulgence in sensuous pleasures. Why do you ask for sensuous pleasures? Why does the mind constantly think about indulgence? Why do you move again and again in the same pattern of indulgences?

For Patanjali, and for all those who have known, the reason is that you are not blissful inwardly, hence the desire for pleasure. The pleasure-oriented mind means that as you are, in yourself, you are unhappy. That's why you seek happiness somewhere else. A person who is unhappy is bound to move into desires. Desires are the way for the unhappy mind to seek happiness. Of course, nowhere can this mind find happiness. At the most he can find a few glimpses; those glimpses appear as pleasure. Pleasure means glimpses of happiness. And the fallacy is that this pleasure-seeking mind thinks that these glimpses and the pleasure are coming from somewhere else. It always comes from within.

Let us try to understand. You are in love with a person, you move into sex. Sex gives you a glimpse of pleasure, it gives you a glimpse of happiness. For a single moment you feel at ease. All the miseries have disappeared, all the mental agony is gone. For a single moment you are here and now, you have forgotten all. For a single moment there is no past and no future – *because* of this there is no past and no future. And for a single moment you are here and now; from within you the energy flows. Your inner self flows in this moment and you have a glimpse of happiness.

But you think that the glimpse is coming from the partner, from the woman or from the man. It is not coming from the man or from the woman, it is coming from you! The other has simply helped you to fall into the present, to fall out of future and past. The other has simply helped to bring you to the nowness of this moment.

If you can come to this nowness without sex, sex by and by will become useless, it will disappear. Then it will not be a desire. If you want to move in it you can move into it as fun, but not as a desire. Then there is no obsession in it because you are not dependent on it.

Sit under a tree some day, just in the morning when the sun has not risen and watch what happens in your body – because with the sun's rising your body is disturbed and it is difficult to be at peace within. That is why in the East they have always been meditating before sunrise. They have called it *brahmamuhurt*, the moments of the divine. And they are right, because with the sun, energies rise and they start flowing in the old pattern that you have created.

Just in the morning, the sun has not yet come on the horizon, everything is silent and nature is fast asleep: the trees are asleep, the birds are asleep, the whole world is asleep; your body also inside is asleep. You have come to sit under a tree. Everything is silent. Just try to be here in this moment. Don't do anything, don't even meditate, don't make any effort. Just close your eyes, remain silent in this silence of nature. Suddenly you will have the same glimpse which has been coming to you through sex or even greater, deeper. Suddenly you will feel a rush of energy flowing from within. And now you cannot be deceived because there is no "other"; it is certainly coming from you, it is certainly flowing from within. Nobody else is giving it to you, you are giving it to yourself.

But the right situation is needed, a silence, energy not in excitement, not doing anything, just being there under a tree. Then you will have the glimpse and this will not really be pleasure, it will be happiness, because now you are looking at the right source, the right direction. Once you know it then through sex you will immediately recognize that the other was just a mirror; you were reflected in him or in her. And you were the mirror for the other. You were helping each other to fall into the present, to move away from the thinking mind to a non-thinking state of being.

The more mind is filled with chattering, the more sex has appeal. In the East sex was never such an obsession as it has become in the West. Films, stories, novels, poetry, magazines, everything has become sexual. You cannot sell anything unless you can create a sex appeal. If you have to sell a car you can sell it only as a sex object. If you want to sell toothpaste you can sell only through some sex appeal. Nothing can be sold without sex. It seems that only sex has the market, nothing else has this significance.

Every significance comes through sex, the whole mind is obsessed with sex. Why? Why has this never happened before? This is something new in human history. And the reason is now the West is totally absorbed in thoughts with no possibility of being here and now, except in sex. Sex has remained the only possibility, and even that is going.

For the modern man it has even become possible that while making love he can think of other things. And once you become so capable that while making love you can go on thinking of something – your bank accounts, talking with a friend, or being somewhere else while making love here – sex will also be finished. Then it will just be boring, frustrating, because sex was not the thing. The thing was only this: that because sexual energy is moving so fast your mind comes to a stop, the sex takes over. The energy flows so fast, so vitally, that your ordinary patterns of thinking stop.

I have heard...

Once it happened that Mulla Nasruddin was passing through a forest. He came upon a skull. Just curious, as he always was, he asked the skull, "What brought you here, sir?"

And he was amazed because the skull said, "Talking brought me here, sir."

He couldn't believe it, but he had heard it so he ran to the court of the king. He told them there, "I have seen a miracle! A skull, a talking skull, lying just near our village in the forest!"

The king also couldn't believe, but he was curious. The whole court followed. They went into the forest. Nasruddin went near the skull and asked again the same question, "What brought you here, sir?" But the skull remained silent. He asked again and again and again, but the skull was dead silent.

The king said, "I knew before, Nasruddin, that you are a liar. But now this is too much. You have played such a joke that you will have to suffer for it." He ordered his guard to cut off his head and throw the head near the skull for the ants to eat. When everybody went – the king, his court – the skull started talking again. And he asked, "What brought you here, sir?"

Nasruddin answered, "What brought me here? Talking brought me here, sir."

Talking has brought man to this situation that is today. A constant chattering mind does not allow any happiness, any possibility of happiness, because only a silent mind can look within, only a silent mind can hear the silence, the happiness that is always bubbling there. But it is so subtle that with the noise of the mind you cannot hear it.

Only in sex the noise sometimes stops. I say sometimes, because if you have become habitual in sex also, as husbands and wives become, then it never stops. The whole act becomes automatic and the mind goes on on its own. Then sex is also a boredom.

Anything has appeal if it can give you a glimpse. The glimpse may appear to be coming from the outside; it always comes from within. The outside can only be just a mirror. When happiness flowing from within is reflected from the outside, it is called pleasure. This is Patanjali's definition: happiness flowing from within reflected from somewhere in the outside, the outside functioning as a mirror. And if you think that this happiness is coming from the outside, it is called pleasure. We are in search of happiness, not in search of pleasure, so unless you can have glimpses of happiness you cannot stop your pleasure-seeking efforts. Indulgence means the search for pleasure.

A conscious effort is needed for two things. One, whenever you feel there is a moment of pleasure, transform it into a meditative situation. Whenever you feel you are feeling pleasure, happy, joyful, close your eyes and look within at where it is coming from. Don't lose this moment, this is precious. If you are not conscious you may continue thinking that it comes from without, and that's the fallacy of the world.

If you are conscious, meditative, if you search for the real source, sooner or later you will come to know it is flowing from within. Once you know that it always flows from within, it is something that you have already got, indulgence will drop, and this will be the first step of desirelessness. Then you are not seeking, not hankering. You are not killing desires, you are not fighting with desires, you have simply found something greater. The desires don't look so important now, they wither away.

Remember this: they are not to be killed and destroyed, they wither away. You simply neglect them because you have a greater source, you are magnetically attracted towards it. Now your whole energy is moving inwards.

The desires are simply neglected. You are not fighting them. If you fight with them you will never win. It is just like you had some stones, colored stones, in your hand and now suddenly you have come to know about diamonds – and they are lying about. You throw away the colored stones just to create space for the diamonds in your hand. You are not fighting the stones. When there are diamonds you simply drop the stones, they have lost their meaning.

Desires must lose their meaning. If you fight, the meaning is not lost. Or even, on the contrary, just through fight you may give them more meaning. Then they become more important. This is happening. Those who fight with any desire, that desire becomes the center of their mind. If you fight sex, sex becomes the center. Then you are continuously engaged, occupied with it. It becomes like a wound. And wherever you look that wound immediately projects, and whatsoever you see becomes sexual.

Mind has a mechanism, an old survival mechanism, of fight or flight. The ways of the mind are two: either you can fight with something or you can escape. If you are strong then you fight, if you are weak then you take flight, then you simply escape, but in both ways the other is important, the other is the center. You can fight or you can escape from the world, from the world where desires are possible. You can go to the Himalayas: that too is a fight, the fight of the weak.

I have heard...

Once Mulla Nasruddin was shopping in a village. He left his donkey on the street and went into a shop to purchase something. When he came out he was furious. Someone had painted his donkey completely red, bright red. So he was furious, and he inquired, "Who has done this? I will kill that man!"

A small boy was standing there. He said, "A man has done this, and that man has just gone inside the pub."

So Nasruddin went there, rushed there, angry, mad. He said, "Who has done this? Who the hell has painted my donkey?"

A very big man, very strong, stood and he said, "I did. What about it?"

So Nasruddin said, "Thank you, sir. You have done such a beautiful job. I just came to tell you that the first coat is dry."

If you are strong then you are ready to fight. If you are weak then you are ready to flee, to take flight. But in both cases you are not becoming stronger. In both cases the other has become the center of your mind. These are the two attitudes, fight or flight – and both are wrong because through both the mind is strengthened.

Patanjali says there is a third possibility: don't fight and don't escape, just be alert. Just be conscious. Whatsoever is the case, just be a witness. Conscious effort means first, searching for the inner source of happiness, and second, witnessing the old pattern of habits, not fighting it, just witnessing it.

> *The first state of vairagya, desirelessness: cessation*
> *from self-indulgence in the thirst for sensuous*
> *pleasures, with conscious effort.*

Conscious effort is the key. Consciousness is needed, and effort is also needed. And the effort should be conscious, because there can be unconscious efforts. You can be trained in such a way that you can drop certain desires without knowing that you have dropped them.

For example, if you are born in a vegetarian home you will be eating vegetarian food. Non-vegetarian food is simply not the question. You never dropped it consciously; you have been brought up in such a way that unconsciously it has dropped by itself. But this is not going to give you some integrity, this is not going to give you some spiritual strength. Unless you do something consciously, it is not gained.

Many societies have tried this for their children, to bring them up in such a way that certain wrong things simply don't enter into their lives. They don't enter, but nothing is gained through it because the real thing to gain is consciousness. And consciousness can be gained through effort. If something is conditioned on you without your effort, it is not a gain at all.

So in India there are many vegetarians. Jainas, brahmins, many people are vegetarians. Nothing is gained because being a vegetarian just by being born in a Jaina family means nothing. It is not a conscious effort, you have not done anything about it. If you were born in a non-vegetarian family you would have taken to non-vegetarian food in the same way.

Unless some conscious effort is done your crystallization never happens. You have to do something on your own. When you do something on your own you gain something. Nothing is gained without consciousness, remember it. It is one of the ultimates – nothing is gained without consciousness! You may become a perfect saint, but if you have not become through consciousness it is futile, useless. You must struggle, inch by inch, because through struggle more consciousness will be needed. And the more consciousness you practice the more conscious you become. And a moment comes when you become pure consciousness.

The first step is:

> ...cessation from self-indulgence in the thirst for sensuous pleasures, with conscious effort.

What to do? Whenever you are in any state of pleasure – sex, food, money, power, anything that gives you pleasure – meditate on it. Just try to find where it is coming from. Are you the source, or is the source somewhere else? If the source is somewhere else then there is no possibility of any transformation because you will remain dependent on the source.

But fortunately, the source is not anywhere else, it is within you. If you meditate you will find it. It is knocking from within every moment, "I am here!" Once you have the feeling that it is there knocking every moment, and you were only creating situations outside in which it was happening, it can happen without situations. Then you need not depend on anybody, not on food, on sex, on power, on anything. You are enough unto yourself. Once you have come to this feeling, the feeling of enoughness, indulgence – the mind that indulges, the indulgent mind – disappears.

That doesn't mean you will not enjoy food. You will enjoy more, but now food is not the source of your happiness, you are the source. You are not dependent on food, you are not addicted to it.

That doesn't mean you will not enjoy sex. You can enjoy more, but now it is fun, play, it is just a celebration. But you are not dependent on it, it is not the source. And once two persons, two lovers, realize that the other is not the source of their pleasure, they stop fighting with the other. They start loving the other for the first time.

You cannot love a person upon whom you are dependent in any way. You will hate, because he is your dependence. Without him you cannot be happy. So he has the key, and a person who has the key to your happiness is your jailer. Lovers fight because they see that the other has the key and, "He can make me happy or unhappy." Once you come to know that you are the source, and the other is the source of his own happiness... You can share your happiness, that's another thing, but you are not dependent. You can share, you can celebrate together. That's what love means: celebrating together, sharing together, not deriving from each other, not exploiting each other, because exploitation cannot be love. Then you are using the other as a means, and whomsoever you use as a means will hate you.

Lovers hate each other because they are using, exploiting each other. And love, which should be the deepest ecstasy, becomes the ugliest hell. But once you know that you are the source of your happiness, no one else is the source, you can share it freely. Then the other is not your enemy, not even an intimate enemy. For the first time friendship arises, you can enjoy anything.

You will be able to enjoy only when you are free. Only an independent person can enjoy. A person who is mad and obsessed with food cannot enjoy. He may fill his belly, but he cannot enjoy. His eating is violent, it is a sort of killing. He is killing the food, he is destroying the food. And lovers who feel that their happiness depends on the other are fighting, trying to dominate the other, trying to kill the other, to destroy the other. You will be able to enjoy everything more when you know that the source is within. Then the whole life becomes a play and moment to moment you can go on celebrating, infinitely.

This is the first step: with effort, consciousness and effort, you achieve desirelessness. Patanjali says this is the first, because even effort, even consciousness is not good because it means some struggle, some hidden struggle, is still on.

The second and last step of *vairagya*, the last state of desire-lessness:

> *...cessation of all desiring by knowing the innermost*
> *nature of purush, the supreme self.*

First, you have to know that you are the source of all happiness that happens to you. Second, you have to know the total nature of your inner self. First, you are the source. Second, "What is this source?" First, just this much is enough – that you are the source of your happiness. And second, what this source is in its totality, what this *purush*, this inner self is – "Who am I?" – in its totality.

Once you know this source in its totality you have known all. Then the whole universe is within. Not only happiness, all that exists, exists within, not only happiness. Then God is not somewhere sitting in the clouds, he exists within. Then you are the source, the root source of all. Then you are the center.

And once you become the center of existence, once you know that you are the center of existence, all misery has disappeared. Now desirelessness becomes spontaneous, *sahaj*. No effort, no striving, no maintaining is needed. It is so; it has become natural. You are not pulling it or pushing it. Now there is no "I" who can pull and push.

Remember this: struggle creates ego. If you struggle in the world it creates a gross ego: "I am someone with money, with pres-tige, with power." If you struggle within it creates a subtle ego: "I am pure, I am a saint, I am a sage" – but "I" remains with struggle. So there are pious egoists who have a very subtle ego. They may not be worldly people – they are not, they are other-worldly – but there is struggle. They have achieved something: that achievement still carries the last shadow of "I."

The second step, and the final state of desirelessness for Patanjali, is total disappearance of the ego: just nature flowing, no "I," no conscious effort. That doesn't mean you will not be conscious; you will be perfect consciousness, but no effort implied of being conscious. There will be no self-consciousness. Pure consciousness means you have accepted yourself and existence as it is.

A total acceptance: this is what Lao Tzu calls Tao, the river flowing towards the sea. It is not making any effort, it is not in any hurry to reach the sea. Even if it doesn't reach it will not get frustrated. Even if it reaches in millions of years, everything is okay. The river is simply flowing because flowing is its nature. There is no effort, it will go on flowing.

When for the first time desires are noted and observed, effort arises, a subtle effort. Even the first step is a subtle effort. You start trying to be aware: "Where is my happiness coming from?" You have to do something, and that doing will create the ego. That's why Patanjali says that is only the beginning, and you must remember that is not the end. In the end not only have desires disappeared, you also have disappeared. Only the inner being has remained in its flow.

This spontaneous flow is the supreme ecstasy, because no misery is possible for it. Misery comes through expectation, demand. There is no one to expect, to demand, so whatsoever happens is good. Whatsoever happens is a blessing. You cannot compare with anything else – it is the case. And because there is no comparing with the past and with the future – there is no one to compare – you cannot look at anything as misery, as pain. Even if pain happens in that situation it will not be painful. Try to understand this. This is difficult.

Jesus is being crucified. Christians have painted Jesus very sad. They have even said that he never laughed, and in their churches they have the sad figure of Jesus everywhere. This is human, we can understand it because a person who is being crucified must be sad, he must be in inner agony, he must be in suffering.

So Christians say that Jesus suffered for our sins – but he suffered. This is absolutely wrong! If you ask Patanjali or me, this is absolutely wrong. Jesus cannot suffer. It is impossible for Jesus to suffer. And if he suffers then there is no difference between you and him.

Pain is there, but he cannot suffer. This may look mysterious, but this is not; this is simple. Pain is there. As far as we can see from the outside he is being crucified, insulted, his body is destroyed. Pain is there but Jesus cannot suffer because in this moment when Jesus is crucified, he cannot ask. He has no demand. He cannot say, "This is wrong. This should not be so. I must be crowned and I am crucified."

If he has in his mind that "I must be crowned and I am crucified," then there will be pain. If he has no "futuring" in his mind that, "I should be crowned," no expectation for the future, no fixed goal to reach, wherever he has found himself is then the goal. And he cannot compare. This cannot be otherwise. This is the present moment that has been brought to him. This crucifixion is the crown.

And he cannot suffer because suffering means resistance. You must resist something, only then can you suffer. Try it. It will be difficult for you to be crucified, but there are daily crucifixions, small ones, but they will do.

You have a pain in the leg, or in the head you have a headache. You may not have observed the mechanism of it: you have a headache and you constantly struggle and resist. You don't want it. You are against it, you divide. You are somewhere standing within the head and the headache is there. You are separate and the headache is separate. You insist that it should not be so, and this is the real problem.

Try once not to fight, flow with the headache, become the headache. And say, "This is the case. This is how my head is at this moment, and at this moment nothing is possible. It may go away in the future, but in this moment the headache is there." Don't resist. Allow it to happen, become one with it. Don't pull yourself separate, flow into it. And then there will be a sudden upsurge of a new type of happiness that you have not known. When there is no one to resist, even a headache is not painful. The fight creates the pain. The pain means always fighting against the pain – that's the real pain.

Jesus accepts: this is how his life has led to the cross. This is the destiny. This is what in the East they have always called fate, *bhagya,* the kismet. So there is no point in arguing with your fate, there is no point in fighting it. You cannot do anything, it is happening. Only one possibility is there for you – you can flow with it or you can fight with it. If you fight it becomes more agony. If you flow with it the agony is less. And if you can flow totally, agony disappears. You become the flow.

Try it when you have a headache, try it when you have an ill body, try it when you have some pain – just flow with it. And if you can allow, you will come to one of the deepest secrets of life: that pain disappears if you flow with it. And if you can flow totally, pain becomes happiness.

But this is not something logical to be understood. You can comprehend it intellectually, but that won't do. Try it existentially. There are everyday situations, every moment something is wrong. Flow with it, and see how you transform the whole situation. And through that transformation you transcend it.

A Buddha can never be in pain, that is impossible. Only an ego can be in pain. To be in pain, ego is a must. And if the ego is there you can also transform your pleasures into pain; if the ego is not there you can transform your pains into pleasures. The secret lies with the ego.

The last state of vairagya, desirelessness: cessation of all desiring by knowing the innermost nature of purush, the supreme self.

How does it happen? – just by knowing the innermost core of yourself, the *purush*, the dweller within. Just by knowing it! Patanjali says, Buddha says, Lao Tzu says, just by knowing it all desires disappear.

This is mysterious, and the logical mind is bound to ask how it can happen that just by knowing themselves all desires disappear. It happens, because not knowing themselves all desires have arisen. Desires are simply the ignorance of the self. Why? All that you are seeking through desires is there, hidden in the self. If you know the self, desires will disappear.

For example, you are asking for power. Everybody is asking for power. Power creates madness in everybody. It seems to be just human: society has existed in such a way that everybody is power-addicted.

The child is born helpless, and this is the first feeling all of you carry with you always. The child is born, he is helpless, and a helpless child wants power. That's natural because everybody is more powerful than he is. The mother is powerful, the father is powerful, the brothers are powerful, everybody is powerful, and the child is absolutely helpless. Of course the first desire that arises is to have power, to grow powerful, to be dominating. And the child starts being political from that very moment. He starts learning the tricks of how to dominate.

If he cries too much he comes to know that he can dominate through crying. He can dominate the whole house just by crying. He learns crying. And women continue it even when they are no longer children. The child has learned the secret and he continues it. And he has to continue it because he remains helpless – that's power politics.

He knows a trick, he can create a disturbance, and he can create such a disturbance that you have to accept and compromise with him. And every moment he feels deeply that the only thing that is needed is power, more power. He will learn, he will go to school, he will grow, he will love, but behind everything – his education, love, play – he will be finding out how to get more power. Through education he will want to dominate, to come first in his class so he can be dominating; to get more money so he can be dominating, to go on growing in influence and the territory of domination. His whole life he will be after power.

Many lives are simply wasted. And even if you get power, what are you going to do? Simply a childish wish is fulfilled. So when you become a Napoleon or a Hitler, suddenly you become aware that the whole effort has been useless, futile. Just a childish wish has been fulfilled, that's all. Now what to do? What to do with this power? If the wish is fulfilled you are frustrated, if the wish is not fulfilled you are frustrated. And it cannot be fulfilled absolutely, because no one can be so powerful that he can feel, "Now it is enough" – no one! The world is so complex that even a Hitler feels powerless in moments, even a Napoleon will feel powerless in moments. Nobody can feel absolute power, and nothing can satisfy you.

But when one comes to know one's self, one comes to know the source of absolute power. Then the desire for power disappears because you were already a king and you were only thinking that you were a beggar. And you were struggling to be a bigger beggar, a greater beggar, and you were already a king. Suddenly you come to realize that you don't lack anything. You are not helpless. You are the source of all energies; you are the very source of life. That childhood feeling of powerlessness was created by others. And it is a vicious circle they created in you because it was created in them by their parents, and so on and so forth.

Your parents are creating the feeling in you that you are powerless.

Why? Because only through this can they feel powerful. You may be thinking that you love children very much. That doesn't seem to be the case. You love power, and when you get children, when you become mothers and fathers, you are powerful. Nobody may be listening to you, you may be nothing in the world, but at least in the boundaries of your home you are powerful. You can at least torture small children.

Look how fathers and mothers torture! And they torture in such a loving way that you cannot even say to them, "You are torturing!" They are torturing, "For their own good" – for the children's own good! They are helping them to grow. They feel powerful. Psychologists say that many people go into the teaching profession just to feel powerful, because with thirty children at your disposal you are just a king.

It is reported that Aurangzeb was imprisoned by his son. When he was imprisoned he wrote a letter and he said, "If you can fulfill only one wish it will be good, and I will be very happy. Just send thirty children to me so that I can teach them in my imprisonment."

The son is reported to have said, "My father has always remained a king, and he cannot lose his kingdom. So even in the prison he needs thirty children so he can teach them."

Look! Go into any school! The teacher sitting on his chair has absolute power, just the master of everything that is happening there. People want children not because they love, because if they really loved the world would be totally different. If you loved your child the world would be totally different. You would not help him to be helpless, to feel helpless. You would give him so much love that he would feel he is powerful. If you give love then he will never be asking for power. He will not become a political leader, he will not try to get elected to anything. He will not try to accumulate money and go mad after it, because he knows it is useless – he is already powerful; love is enough. But nobody is giving love, so he will create substitutes.

All your desires, whether for power, money, prestige, all show that something had been taught to you in your childhood, something has been conditioned in your biocomputer, and you are following that conditioning without looking inside to find that whatsoever you are asking for is already there.

Patanjali's whole effort is to put your biocomputer into silence so that it doesn't interfere. This is what meditation is. It is putting your biocomputer, for certain moments, into silence, into a non-chattering state, so you can look within and hear your deepest nature. Just a glimpse will change you because then this biocomputer cannot deceive you. This biocomputer goes on saying, "Do this, do that!" It goes on continuously manipulating you: "You must have more power, otherwise you are nobody."

If you look within, there is no need to be anybody. There is no need to be somebody. You are already accepted as you are. The whole existence accepts you, is happy about you. You are a flowering, an individual flowering, different from any other, unique. And God welcomes you, otherwise you could not be here. You are here only because you are accepted. You are here only because God loves you or the universe loves you or existence needs you. You are needed.

Once you know your innermost nature, what Patanjali calls the *purush* – *purush* means the inner dweller, the body is just a house, the inner dweller, the inner-dwelling consciousness, is *purush* – once you know this inner-dwelling consciousness, nothing is needed. You are enough, more than enough, you are perfect as you are. You are absolutely accepted, welcomed. The existence becomes a blessing. Desires disappear; they were part of self-ignorance. With self-knowledge they disappear, they evaporate.

Abhyasa, constant inner practice, conscious effort to be more and more alert, to be more and more master of oneself, to be less and less dominated by habits, by mechanical, robot-like mechanisms, and *vairagya*, desirelessness: these two attained, one becomes a yogi. These two attained, one has attained the goal.

I will repeat: don't create a fight. Allow all this happening to be more and more spontaneous. Don't fight with the negative. Rather, create the positive. Don't fight with sex, with food, with anything. Rather, find out what it is that gives you happiness, from where it comes; move in that direction. Desires, by and by, go on disappearing.

And be more and more conscious. Whatsoever is happening, be more and more conscious. And remain in that moment and accept that moment. Don't ask for something else. Then you will not be creating misery. If pain is there, let it be there. Remain in it and flow in it. The only condition is, remain alert. Knowingly, watchfully, move into it, flow into it, don't resist.

When pain disappears the desire for pleasure also disappears. When you are not in anguish you don't ask for indulgence. When anguish is not there indulgence becomes meaningless, and you go on falling into the inner abyss more and more. And it is so blissful, it is such a deep ecstasy, that even a glimpse of it and the whole world becomes meaningless. Then all that this world can give to you is of no use.

This should not become a fighting attitude. You should not become a warrior, you should become a meditator. If you are meditating, spontaneously things will happen to you which will go on transforming and changing you. Start fighting and you have started suppression. And suppression will lead you into more and more misery.

And you cannot deceive. There are many people who are not only deceiving others, they are deceiving themselves. They think they are not in misery. They go on saying they are not in misery but their whole existence is miserable. When they are saying that they are not in misery their faces, their eyes, their heart, everything, is in misery. I will tell you one anecdote, and then finish.

I have heard...

Once it happened that twelve ladies reached purgatory. The officiating angel asked them, "Were any of you unfaithful to your husbands while on earth? If someone was unfaithful to her husband, she should raise her hand." Blushingly, hesitating, by and by, eleven ladies raised their hands.

The officiating angel took his phone, called into the phone, "Hello! Is that hell? Have you got room for twelve unfaithful wives there? – One of them, stone deaf!"

It isn't needed for you to say it or not – your face, your very being, shows everything. You may say you are not miserable but the way you say it, the way you are, shows you are miserable. You cannot deceive. And there is no point because no one can deceive anybody else, you can only deceive yourself.

Remember, if you are miserable, you have created all this. Let it penetrate deep into your heart that you have created your sufferings, because this is going to be the formula, the key. If you have created your sufferings, only then can you destroy them. If someone else has created them, you are helpless. You have created your miseries; you can destroy them. You have created them through wrong habits, wrong attitudes, addictions, desires.

Drop this pattern. Look afresh, and this very life is the ultimate joy that is possible to human consciousness.

Enough for today.

CHAPTER 10

the end is in the beginning

The first question:

> Osho,
> How is it that you describe the life that is really ours, and
> which you have transcended, so correctly and in every
> detail, while we remain so ignorant of it? Is it not
> paradoxical?

It looks paradoxical; it is not. But you can understand only when
you have transcended. While you are in a certain state of mind you
cannot understand that state of mind; you are so involved in it,
you are so identified with it. For understanding, space is needed,
a distance is needed; and there is no distance. When you transcend a
state of mind, only then you become able to understand it because
then there is distance. You are standing aloof, separate. Now you can
look, unidentified. Now there is perspective.

While you are in love you cannot understand love. You may feel
it but you cannot understand it. You are too much in it, and for
understanding, an aloofness, detached aloofness is needed. For understanding, you need to be an observer. While you are in love the

observer is lost, you have become a doer. You are a lover, you cannot be a witness to it. Only when you transcend love, when you are enlightened and have gone beyond love, will you be able to understand it.

A child cannot understand what childhood is. When childhood is lost you can look back and understand. Youth cannot understand what youth is. Only when you have become old and are capable of looking back with aloofness, distance, will you be able to understand it. Whatsoever is understood, is understood only by transcendence. Transcendence is the base of all understanding. That's why it happens every day: you can give advice, good advice, to somebody else who is in trouble; if you are in the same trouble you cannot give that good advice to yourself.

Somebody else is in trouble, you have space to look, observe; you can witness. You can give good advice. When you are in the same trouble you will not be so capable. You can be, if even then you can be detached. You can be, if even then you can look at the problem as if you are not in the problem, but outside, standing on a hill and looking down.

Any problem can be solved if even for a single moment you are out of it and can look at it as a witness. Witnessing solves everything. But while you are deep in any state it is difficult to be a witness because you are so much identified. While in anger you become anger. No one is left behind who can see, observe, watch, decide. No one is left behind. While in sex you have moved completely, now there is no uninvolved center.

In the Upanishads it is said that a person who is watching himself is like a tree upon which two birds are sitting: one bird just jumping, enjoying, eating, singing, and the other bird just sitting on the top of the tree looking at the first bird.

If you can have a witnessing self on the top which goes on looking at the drama below, where you are the actor, where you participate, dance and jump and sing and talk and think and get involved; if somebody deep in you can go on looking at this drama, if you can be in a state where you are playing as an actor on the stage and simultaneously sitting in the audience looking at it; if you can be the actor and the audience both, then witnessing has come in. This witnessing will make you capable of knowing, of understanding, of wisdom.

So it looks paradoxical. If you go to Buddha he can move into deep details of your problems not because he is in the problem, only because he is not in the problem. He can penetrate you. He can put himself in your situation and still remain a witness.

So those who are in the world cannot understand the world. Only those who have gone beyond it can understand it. So whatsoever you want to understand, go beyond it. This appears paradoxical. Whatsoever you want to know, go beyond it; only then will knowledge happen. Moving as an insider in anything you may collect much information, but you will not become a wise man.

You can practice it moment to moment. You can do both: be the actor and be the audience. When you are angry you can shift the mind. This is a deep art, but if you try you will be able; you can shift.

For a single moment you can be angry. Then get detached, look at the anger, at your own face in the mirror. Look at what you are doing, look at what is happening around you, look at what you have done to others and how they are reacting. Look for a moment, then again allow the anger, move into the anger. Then again become an observer. This can be done, but then very deep practice is needed.

Try it. While eating, for one moment become the eater. Enjoy, become the food, become the eating; forget that there is anyone who can look at it. Then for a single moment move away. Go on eating but start looking at the food, the eater, and you standing above looking at it.

Soon you will become efficient and you can shift the gears of the mind from the actor to the audience, from the participant to the onlooker. And then this will be revealed to you: that through participation nothing is known. Only through observation do things become revealed and known. That's why those who have left the world have become the guides. Those who have gone beyond have become the masters.

Freud used to say to his disciples... It is very difficult, because Freud's disciples, the psychoanalysts, are not men who have transcended. They live in the world, they are just experts. But even Freud has suggested to them that while listening to a patient, to someone who is ill, mentally ill, "Remain detached. Don't get emotionally involved. If you get involved then your advice is futile. Just remain a spectator."

It looks very cruel. Somebody is crying, weeping, and you can also feel sad because you are a human being. But Freud said, "If you are working as a psychiatrist, as a psychoanalyst, remain uninvolved. Look at the person as if he is just a problem. Don't look at him as if he is a human being. If you look at him as a human being you are immediately involved, you have become a participant; then you cannot advise. Then whatsoever you say will be prejudiced. Then you are not outside it."

It is difficult, very difficult, so Freudians have been doing it through many ways. The Freudian psychoanalyst will not face the patient directly, because when you face a person it is difficult to remain uninvolved. If you look in the eyes of a person, you enter him. So the Freudian psychoanalyst sits behind a curtain and the patient lies on a couch.

That too is very significant, because Freud came to understand that if a person is lying down and you are sitting or standing, not looking at him, there is less possibility to get involved. Why? A person who is lying down becomes "a problem," as if on the surgeon's table; you can dissect him. And ordinarily this never happens. If you go to meet a person he will not talk to you lying down and you sitting unless he is a patient, unless he is in the hospital.

So Freud insists that his patient should lie down on the couch. So the psychoanalyst goes on feeling that the person is a patient, ill; he has to be helped. He is not really a person but a problem, and you need not get involved with him. Also the psychoanalyst should not face the patient but listen to him while hiding behind a curtain. Freud says don't touch the patient, because if you touch, if you take the patient's hand in your hand, there is a possibility you may get involved.

These precautions have been taken because psychoanalysts are not enlightened persons. But if you go to a buddha there is no need for you to lie down, there is no need for a curtain. There is no need for a buddha to remain conscious so that he does not get involved; he *cannot* get involved. Whatsoever the case, he remains uninvolved.

He can feel compassion for you but he cannot be sympathetic, remember this. And try to understand the distinction between sympathy and compassion. Compassion is from a higher source. A buddha can remain compassionate towards you. He understands you, that you are in a difficulty, but he is not sympathetic with you because he knows it is because of your foolishness that you are in difficulty, it is your stupidity that you are in difficulty.

He has compassion: he will try in every way to help you to come out of your stupidity, but your stupidity is not something with which he is going to sympathize. So in a way he will be very warm and in a way he will be very cold. He will be warm as far as his compassion is concerned, and he will be absolutely cold as far as sympathy is concerned.

And ordinarily, if you go to a buddha you will feel he is cold because you don't know what compassion is and you don't know the warmth of compassion. You have known only the warmth of sympathy, and he is not sympathetic. He looks cruel, cold. If you cry and weep he is not going to cry and weep with you. And if he cries then there is no possibility that help can come from him to you; he is in the same position. He cannot cry, but you will feel hurt: "I am crying and weeping and he remains just like a statue, as if he has no heart." He cannot sympathize with you. Sympathy is from the same mind towards the same mind, compassion is from a higher source.

He can look at you. You are transparent to him, totally naked. And he knows why you are suffering – you are the cause. And he will try to explain the cause to you, and if you can listen to him the very act of listening will have helped you much.

It looks paradoxical, it is not. A buddha has also lived like you. If not in this life, then in some previous lives he has moved through the same struggles. He has been stupid like you, he has suffered like you, he has struggled like you. For many, many lives he was on the same path. He knows all the agony, all the struggle, the conflict, the misery. He is aware, more aware than you, because now all the past lives are before his eyes, and not only his, but your lives also. He has lived all the problems that any human mind can live, so he knows. And he has transcended them, so now he knows what the causes are and he also knows how they can be transcended.

He will help in every way to make you understand that you are the cause of your miseries. This is very hard. This is the most difficult thing to understand, that "I am the cause of my miseries." This hits deep, one feels hurt. Whenever someone says someone else is the cause you feel okay and that person looks sympathetic. If he says, "You are a sufferer, a victim, and others are exploiting you, others are doing damage, others are violent," you feel good. But this goodness is not going to last. It is a momentary consolation, and dangerous, at a very great cost, because he is helping the cause of your misery.

So those who look sympathetic towards you are really your enemies, because their sympathy helps your cause to be strengthened. The very source of misery is strengthened. You feel that you are okay and the whole world is wrong: misery comes from somewhere else.

If you go to a buddha, to an enlightened person, he is bound to be hard, because he will force you to see the fact that you are the cause. And once you start feeling that you are the cause of your hell, the transformation has already started. The moment you feel this, half the work is already done. You are already on the path, you have already moved. A great change has come over you.

Half the miseries will suddenly disappear once you understand that you are the cause, because then you cannot cooperate. Then you will not be so ignorant to help strengthen the cause which creates miseries. Your cooperation will break. Miseries will still continue for a while just because of old habits.

Mulla Nasruddin was once forced to go to court because he had been found drunk on the street. The magistrate said, "Nasruddin, I remember seeing you so many times for this same offense. Have you got any explanation for your habitual drunkenness?"

Nasruddin said, "Of course, your Honor. I have an explanation for my habitual drunkenness. This is my explanation: habitual thirst."

Even if you become alert, the habitual pattern will force you for a while to move in the same direction. But it cannot persist for long, the energy is no longer there. It may continue as a dead pattern, but by and by it will wither away. It needs to be fed every day, it needs every day to be strengthened. Your cooperation is needed continuously.

Once you become alert that you are the cause of your miseries, the cooperation drops. So whatsoever I say to you is just to make you alert of a single fact: that wherever you are, whatsoever you are, you are the cause. And don't get pessimistic about it, this is very hopeful – if somebody else is the cause then nothing can be done.

Because of this, Mahavira denies God. Mahavira says there is no God, because if there is God then nothing can be done: "Because if *he* is the cause of everything, then what can *I* do? Then I become helpless. He has created the world, he has created me. If he is the creator then only he can destroy. And if I am miserable then he is responsible and I cannot do anything." So Mahavira says, "If there is God then man is helpless." So he says, "I don't believe in God." And the reason is not philosophical, the reason is very psychological. The reason is so that you cannot make anybody responsible for you. Whether God exists or not is not the question.

Mahavira says, "I want you to understand that you are the cause of whatsoever you are." And this is very hopeful. If you are the cause you can change it. If you can create hell, you can create heaven. You are the master.

So don't feel hopeless. The more you make others responsible for your life the more you are a slave. If you say, "My wife is making me angry," then you are a slave. If you say your husband is creating trouble for you, then you are a slave. Even if your husband is creating trouble, you have chosen that husband. And you wanted this trouble, this type of trouble is your choice. If your wife is making hell, remember that you have chosen this wife.

Somebody asked Mulla Nasruddin, "How did you come to know your wife? Who introduced you?"

He said, "It just happened. I cannot blame anybody."

Nobody can blame anybody. And it is not just a happening, it is a choice. A particular type of man chooses a particular type of woman, it is not an accident. And he chooses for particular reasons. If this woman dies he will again choose the same type of woman. If he divorces this woman again he will marry the same type of woman. You can go on changing wives, but unless the husband changes there can be no real change, only names change. Because this man has a choice: he likes a particular face, he likes a particular nose, he likes particular eyes, he likes a particular behavior.

And that's a complex thing. If you like a particular nose...because a nose is not just a nose: it carries anger, it carries ego, it carries silence, it carries peace, it carries many things. If you like a particular nose, you may like a person who can force you to be angry. An egoistic person carries a different type of nose. It may look beautiful only because you are in search of somebody who can create a hell around you. And sooner or later things will follow; you may not be able to connect, you may not be able to link. Life is complex, and you are so much involved in it that you cannot connect. You will be able to see only when you transcend.

It is just like when you fly in an aircraft over and above Mumbai, then the whole of Mumbai appears, the whole pattern. If you live in Mumbai and move in the streets, you cannot look at the whole pattern. The whole of Mumbai cannot be seen by those who live in Mumbai, it can be seen only by those who fly above. Then the whole pattern appears, things fall into a pattern. Transcendence means going beyond human problems. Then you can enter and see.

I have looked through many, many persons. Whatsoever they do, they are not aware of what they are doing. They become aware only when results come. They go on dropping the seed in the soil – they are not aware – only when they will have to reap will they become aware. And they cannot connect that they are the source and they are the reapers.

Once you understand that you are the cause, you have moved onto the path. Now many things become possible. Now you can do something about the problem that is your life. You can change it. Just by changing yourself, you can change.

A woman who belongs to a very rich family, a very good family, cultured, refined, educated, came to me. She asked me, "If I start meditating, will it in any way disturb my relationship with my husband?" And she herself said, before I answered her, "I know it is not going to disturb it because if I become better, more silent and more loving, how can it disturb my relationship?"

But I told her, "You are wrong. The relationship is going to be disturbed. Whether you become good or bad, that is irrelevant. You change – one partner changes – the relationship is going to be disturbed. And this is the miracle: that if you become bad the relationship will not be disturbed so much. If you become good and better the relationship is just going to be shattered, because when one partner falls down and becomes bad, the other feels better, comparatively. It is not a hurt to the ego; rather, it is ego-satisfying."

So a wife feels good if the husband starts drinking, because now she becomes a moral preacher. Now she dominates him more. Now whenever he enters in the house he enters like a criminal. And just because he drinks, everything that he is doing becomes wrong. That much is enough, because the wife can bring that argument again and again from anywhere, so everything is condemned.

But if a husband or a wife becomes meditative, then there will be deeper problems because the other's ego will be hurt. One is becoming superior and the other will try in every way not to allow this to happen. He will create all the troubles possible. And even if it happens he will try not to believe that it has happened. He will prove that this has not happened yet. He will go on saying that, "You are meditating for years and nothing has happened. What is the use of it? Useless! You still get angry, you still do this and that, you remain the same." The other will try to force it that nothing is happening. This is a consolation.

And if *really* something has happened, if the wife or the husband has really changed, then this relationship cannot continue. It is impossible unless the other is also ready to change. And to get ready to change oneself is very difficult because it hurts the ego, it means that whatsoever you are, you are wrong. Only then is a need for change felt.

So nobody ever feels that he has to change: "The whole world has to change, not I. I am the right, the absolute right, and the world is wrong because it doesn't fit to me." All the effort of all the buddhas is very simple: it is to make you aware that wherever you are, whatsoever you are, you are the cause.

The second question:

Osho,
Why do so many persons on the path of Yoga adopt an attitude of fight, struggle, over-concern with keeping strict rules and warrior-like ways? Is this necessary in order to really be a yogi?

It is absolutely unnecessary. Not only unnecessary, it creates all types of hindrances on the path of Yoga. The warrior-like attitude is the greatest hindrance possible because there is no one to fight with. Inside, you are alone. If you start fighting you are splitting yourself.

This is the greatest disease: to be divided, to become schizophrenic. And the whole struggle is useless because it is not going to lead anywhere. No one can win. You are on both sides, so at the most you can play, you can play a game of hide and seek. Sometimes part *A* wins, sometimes part *B* wins, again part *A*, again part *B*. In this way you can move. Sometimes that which you call good wins. But fighting with the bad, winning over the bad, the good part has become exhausted and the bad part has gathered energy. So sooner or later the bad part will come up, and this can go on infinitely.

But why does this warrior-like attitude happen? Why, with most people, does fighting start? The moment they think of transformation they start fighting. Why? – because you know only one method of winning, and that is fight.

In the world outside, in the outside world, there is one way to be victorious and that is fight; fight and destroy the other. This is the only way to be victorious in the outside world. And you have lived in this outside world for millions and millions of years and you have been fighting, sometimes getting defeated if you don't fight well, sometimes being victorious if you fight well. It has become a built-in program to "Fight strongly"; there is only one way to be victorious and that is a hard fight.

When you move within you carry the same program because you are acquainted only with this. And in the world within, just the reverse is the case: fight and you will be defeated, because there is no one to fight with. In the inner world, let-go is the way to be victorious, surrender is the way to be victorious, allowing the inner nature to flow, not fighting, is the way to be victorious. Letting the river flow, not pushing it, is the way as far as the inner world is concerned; this is just the reverse. But you are acquainted only with the outside world, so this is bound to be so in the beginning. Whoever moves within will carry the same weapons, the same attitudes, the same fighting, the same defense.

Machiavelli is for the outside world; Lao Tzu, Patanjali or Buddha are for the inside world. And they teach different things. Machiavelli says attack is the best defense: "Don't wait. Don't wait for the other to attack, because then you are already losing. Already you have lost, because the other has started. He has already gained so it is always better to start. Don't wait to defend, always be the aggressor. Before somebody else attacks you, you attack him. And fight with as much cunningness as possible, with as much dishonesty as possible. Be dishonest, be cunning and be aggressive. Deceive, because that is the only way." These are the means that Machiavelli suggests. And Machiavelli is an honest man, that's why he suggests exactly whatsoever is needed.

But if you ask Lao Tzu, Patanjali or Buddha, they are talking of a different type of victory – the inner victory. There, cunningness won't do, deceiving won't do, fighting won't do, aggression won't do, because whom are you going to deceive? Whom are you going to defeat? You alone are there. In the outside world you are never alone, "the others" are there; they are the enemies. In the inside world you alone are there, there is no other. There is no enemy, no friend. This is a totally new situation for you. You will carry the old weapons, but those old weapons will become the cause of your defeat. When you change the world from without to within, leave all that you have learned from without; that is not going to help.

Somebody asked Ramana Maharshi, "What should I learn to become silent, to know myself?" Ramana Maharshi is reported to have said, "For reaching to the inner self you need not learn anything. You need unlearning. Learning won't help, it helps you to move without. Unlearning will help."

Whatsoever you have learned, unlearn it, forget it, drop it. Move inside innocently, childlike, not with cunningness and cleverness but childlike trust and innocence; not thinking in terms that someone is going to attack you. There is no one, so don't feel insecure and don't make any arrangements for your defense. Remain vulnerable, receptive, open. That's what *shraddha*, trust, means.

Doubt is needed on the outside because the other is there. He may be thinking to deceive you, so you have to doubt and be skeptical. Inside, no doubt, no skepticism is needed. Nobody is there to deceive you, you can remain there just as you are.

That's why everybody carries this warrior-like attitude, but it is not needed. It is a hindrance, the greatest hindrance. Drop it outside. You can make it a point to remember that whatsoever is needed outside will become a hindrance inside – whatsoever, I say, unconditionally. And just the reverse has to be tried.

If doubt helps on the outside, in scientific research, then faith will help on the inside, in religious inquiry. If aggressiveness helps on the outside in the world of power, prestige, others, then non-aggressiveness will help on the inside. If a cunning, calculating mind helps on the outside, then an innocent, non-calculating, childlike mind will help on the inside.

Remember this: whatsoever helps on the outside, just the reverse will do on the inside. So read Machiavelli's *The Prince*; that is

the way for outside victory. And just make a reverse of Machiavelli's
The Prince, and you can reach inside. Just make Machiavelli stand
upside-down and he becomes Lao Tzu – just in *shirshasan*, in the
headstand. Machiavelli standing on his head becomes Patanjali.

So read his book *The Prince*: it is beautiful, the clearest statement for the outside victory. And then read Lao Tzu's *Tao Te Ching*
or Patanjali's *Yoga Sutras* or Buddha's *Dhammapada* or Jesus'
Sermon on the Mount: they are contradictory, just the reverse, just
the opposite.

Jesus says, "Blessed are those who are meek because they will
inherit the earth" – meek, innocent, weak, not strong in any sense –
"Blessed are the poor because they will enter the kingdom of God."
And Jesus makes it clear: "poor in spirit." They have nothing to claim.
They cannot say, "I have got this." They don't possess anything –
knowledge, wealth, power, prestige. They don't possess anything, they
are poor, they cannot claim, "This is mine."

We go on claiming, "This is mine, that is mine. The more I can
claim, the more I feel, 'I am'." In the outside world the greater the
territory of your mind, the more you are. In the inner world the less
the territory of mind, the greater you are. And when the territory disappears completely and you have become a zero, then you are the
greatest. Then you are the victor. Then the victory has happened.

Warrior-like attitudes – struggle, fight, over-concern with strict
rules, regulations, calculations, planning – this mind is carried inside
because you have learned it and you don't know anything else;
hence the necessity of a master. Otherwise you will go on trying
your ways which are absolutely absurd there.

This is why initiation is necessary. Initiation means somebody can
show you the path where you have never traveled; somebody can give
you a glimpse through him of a world, of a dimension, that is absolutely unknown to you. You are almost blind to it. You cannot see it,
because eyes can see only whatsoever they have learned to see.

If you come here and you are a tailor, then you don't look at faces,
you look at dresses. Faces don't mean much; just looking at the
dress you know what type of man is there. You know a language.

If you are a shoemaker you need not even look at the dress, just
shoes will do. And a shoemaker can just go on looking on the street,
just looking at the shoe, and he knows who is passing, whether he is
a great leader or whether he is an artist, a bohemian, a hippie, a rich

man, cultured, educated, uneducated, a villager. He knows who he is just by looking at the shoe, because a shoe gives all the indications. He knows the language. If the man is winning in his life then the shoe has a different shine. If he is defeated in life, the shoe is defeated: then the shoe is sad, not cared for. And the shoemaker knows it. He need not look at your face, the shoe will tell everything that he wants to know.

Everything we learn, we become fixed in it. Then that's what we see. You have learned something, and you have wasted many lives in learning it. And it is now deep-rooted, imprinted; it has become part of your brain cells. So when you move within there is simply darkness, nothing, you cannot see anything. The whole world that you know has disappeared.

It is just like you know one language and suddenly you are transported to a land where no one understands your language and you cannot understand anybody else's language. And people are talking and chattering and you feel that they are simply mad. It looks as if they are talking gibberish, and it looks very noisy because you cannot understand. And they seem to be talking too loudly. If you can understand it then the whole thing changes, you become part of it. Then it is not gibberish, it becomes meaningful.

When you enter within you know the language of the without. There is darkness within. Your eyes cannot see, your ears cannot hear, your hands cannot feel. Somebody is needed, somebody to initiate you, to take your hand in his hand and to move you onto this unknown path until you become acquainted, until you start feeling, until you become aware of some light, some meaning, some signifi-cance around you.

Once you have the first initiation things will start happening. But the first initiation is a difficult thing because this is quite an about-turn, a total about-turn. Suddenly your world of meaning disappears; you are in a strange world. You don't understand anything – where to move, what to do and what to make out of this chaos. A master only means someone who knows. And this chaos, this inside chaos, is not chaos for him; it has become an order, a cosmos, and he can lead you into it.

Initiation means looking into the inner world through someone else's eyes. Without trust it is impossible because you won't allow your hand to be taken, you won't allow anybody to lead you into the unknown. And he cannot give you any guarantee, no guarantee will be of any use. Whatsoever he says, you have to take it on trust.

In the old days, when Patanjali was writing his sutras, trust was very easy, because in the outside world also – particularly in the East and especially in India – they had also created an outside pattern of initiation. For example, trades, professions, belonged to families through heredity. A father would initiate the child into the profession, and a child naturally believes in his father. The father would take the child to the farm if he was a peasant and a farmer, and he would initiate him into his farming. Whatsoever trade, whatsoever business he was doing, he would initiate the child.

In the outside world also, there was initiation in the East. Everything was done by an initiation; someone who knew would take you. This helped very much because you were acquainted with initiation, with someone leading you. So, when the time came for inner initiation, you could trust.

And trust, *shraddha*, faith, was easier in a world which was non-technological. A technological world needs cunning, calculation, mathematics, cleverness; not innocence. In a technological world if you are innocent you will look foolish, if you are cunning you will look clever, intelligent. Our universities are doing nothing but this: they make you clever, cunning, calculating. The more calculating, the more cunning, the more successful you will be in the world.

In the East quite the reverse was the case in the past: if you were cunning it was impossible for you to succeed even in the outside world. Only innocence was accepted. Technique was not valued much but inner quality was valued very much.

In the East, in the past, if a person was cunning and he made a better shoe, nobody would go to him. They would go to the person who was innocent. He might not make such good shoes, but they would go to the person who was innocent because a shoe is not just something, it carries the quality of the person who has made it. So if there was a cunning and clever technician nobody would go to him. He would suffer, he would be a failure. But if he was a man of qualities, of character, of innocence, then people would go to him even for worse things; people would value his things more.

Kabir was a weaver, and he remained a weaver. Even when he attained enlightenment he continued weaving. And he was so ecstatic that his weaving could not have been very good. He was singing and dancing and weaving! There were many mistakes and many errors, but his things were valued, super-valued.

Many people would just wait for Kabir to bring something: that was not just a thing, a commodity, it was from Kabir. The very thing in itself had an intrinsic quality as it had come from Kabir's hands, Kabir had touched it. And Kabir was dancing around it while he was weaving it. And he was continuously remembering the divine, so the thing – the cloth or the dress or anything – had become sacred, holy. The quantity was not the question, but the quality! The technical side was secondary, the human side was primary.

So in the East, even in the outside world they had managed a pattern so that when you turned inward you would not be totally unacquainted with that world. You would know something, you had some guidelines, some lights in your hand. You would not be moving into total darkness.

This trust in outside relationships was everywhere. A husband couldn't believe that his wife could be unfaithful. It was almost impossible. And if the husband died, the wife would die with him because life was such a shared phenomenon. Now it was meaningless to live without someone with whom life had become such a shared thing.

It became ugly later on, but in the beginning it was one of the most beautiful things that has ever happened on earth. You loved someone and he has disappeared; you would like to disappear with him. To be without him would be worse than death. Death was better and worth choosing – such was the trust in outside things also. The relationship of wife and husband is an outside thing. The whole society was moving around trust, faith, authentic sharing. Then it was helpful. When once the time came to move within, all these things would help him to be initiated easily, to trust someone, to surrender.

Fight, struggle, aggressiveness are hindrances. Don't carry them. When you move inward, leave them at the door. If you carry them you will miss the inner temple, you will never reach it. With those things you cannot move inward.

The third question:

Osho,
Is not vairagya, non-attachment or desirelessness,

enough in itself to free one from worldly bondage? What
then is the use of yogic discipline, abhyasa?

Vairagya is enough, desirelessness is enough. Then no discipline
is needed. But where is that desirelessness? It is not there. To help it,
discipline is needed. Discipline is needed only because that desirelessness is not within you in its wholeness.

If desirelessness is there then there is no question of practicing
anything: no discipline is needed. You will not come to listen to me,
you will not go to read Patanjali's sutras. If desirelessness is complete Patanjali is useless. Why waste your time with Patanjali's
sutras? I am useless, why come to me?

You are in search of a discipline. You are moving in search of
some discipline which can transform you. You are a disciple, and
disciple means a person who is in search of a discipline. And don't
deceive yourself – even if you go to Krishnamurti you are in search
of a discipline, because one who is not in need will not go. Even if
Krishnamurti says that no one needs to be a disciple and no discipline is needed, why are you there? These words will become your
discipline, and you will create a pattern and you will start following
that pattern.

Desirelessness is not there, so you are in suffering. And nobody
likes to suffer, and everybody wants to transcend suffering. How to
transcend it? This is what discipline will help you to do. Discipline
only means to make you ready for the jump, for the jump of desirelessness. Discipline means a training.

You are not yet ready. You have a very gross mechanism. Your
body and your mind are gross, they cannot receive the subtle. You are
not tuned. To receive the subtle you will have to be tuned, your gross-
ness has to disappear. Remember this: to receive the subtle you will
have to become subtle. As you are, the divine may be around you but
you cannot be in touch with it.

It is just like a radio lying here in this room but not functioning.
Some wires are wrongly connected, or some wires are broken or some
knob is missing. The radio is here, the radio waves are continuously
passing, but the radio is not tuned and it cannot become receptive.

You are just like a radio that is not in a state where it can function. Many things are missing, many things are wrongly joined. A
discipline means to make your radio functioning, receptive, tuned.

The divine waves are all around you; once you are tuned they become manifest. And they can become manifest only through you, and unless they become manifest through you, you cannot know them. They may have become manifest through me, they may have become manifest through Krishnamurti or anybody else, but that cannot become your transformation.

You cannot really know what is happening in a Krishnamurti, in a Gurdjieff, what is happening inside, what type of tuning is happening, how their mechanism has become so subtle that it receives the subtlest message of the universe, the existence starts manifesting itself through it.

Discipline means to change your mechanism, to tune it, to make it a fit instrument to be expressive, receptive. Sometimes without discipline this can also accidentally happen. The radio can fall from the table. Just by falling, just by accident, some wires may get connected or disconnected. Just by falling the radio may get connected to a station. Then it will start expressing something, but it will be a chaos.

It has happened many times. Sometimes through accident people have come to know the divine and feel the divine. But then they go mad because they are not disciplined to receive such a great phenomenon. They are not ready. They are so small, and such a great ocean falls in them. This has happened. In the Sufi system they call such persons "madmen of God," they call them *masts*.

Many people, through some accident, through some master, through the grace of some master or just through the presence of some master, get tuned sometimes without discipline. Their whole mechanism is not ready but a part starts functioning. Then they are out of order. Then you will feel they are mad, because they will start saying things which look irrelevant. And they can also feel that they are irrelevant, but they cannot do anything. Something has begun in them, they cannot stop it. They feel a certain happiness. That's why they are called *masts*, the happy ones. But they are not buddha-like, they are not enlightened. And it is said that for *masts*, for these happy ones who have gone mad, a very great master is needed because now they cannot do anything with themselves. They are just in confusion – happily in it, but they are a mess. And now they cannot do anything on their own.

In the old days great Sufi masters would move all around the earth. They would go whenever they heard that somewhere there was a *mast*, a madman; they would go and they would just help that man to get tuned.

In this century only Meher Baba has done that work – a great work of its own type, a rare work. Continuously, for many years, he traveled all over India, and the places he visited were madhouses, because many *masts* are living in madhouses. But you cannot make any distinction, who is mad and who is *mast* – they are both mad. Who is really mad and who is mad just because of a divine accident, because of some tuning that has happened through some accident? You cannot make any distinction.

There are many *masts*. Meher Baba traveled and he would live in the madhouses, and he would help and serve the *masts*, the mad ones. And many of them came out of their madness and started their journey toward enlightenment.

In the West many people are in madhouses, mad asylums, many who don't need any psychiatric help, because psychiatrists can only make them normal again. They need the help of someone who is enlightened, not a psychiatrist. Because they are not ill, or if they are ill, they are ill by a divine disease. Your health is nothing before that illness. That illness is better, worth losing all your health for. Discipline is needed.

In India, this phenomenon has not been as great as it has been in Mohammedan countries. That's why Sufis have special methods to help *mast* people, the mad people of God.

But Patanjali has created such a subtle system that there is no need of any accident. The discipline is so scientific that if you pass through this discipline you will reach to buddhahood without going mad on the path. It is a complete system.

Sufism is still not a complete system. Many things are lacking in it, and they are lacking because of the stubborn attitude of Mohammedans. They won't allow it to evolve to its peak and climax. And the Sufi system has to follow the pattern of the Islamic religion. Because of the structure of the Mohammedan religion, the Sufi system couldn't go beyond.

Patanjali follows no religion, he follows only truth. He will not make any compromise with Hinduism or Mohammedanism or any "ism." He follows the scientific truth. Sufis had to make compromises – they *had* to. Because there were some Sufis who tried not to make any compromise, for example, Bayazid of Bistham or al-Hillaj

Mansur who didn't make any compromise and they were killed, they were murdered.

So Sufis went into hiding. They made their science completely secret and they allowed only fragments to be known – only those fragments which fit with Islam and its pattern. All other fragments were hidden. So the whole system is not known; it is not working. So many people, through fragments, go mad.

Patanjali's system is complete, and discipline is needed. Before you move into this unknown world of the within, a deep discipline is needed so no accident is possible. If you move without discipline, then many things are possible.

Vairagya is enough, but that "enough *vairagya*" is not there in your heart. If it is there, then there is no question. Then close Patanjali's book and burn it; it is absolutely unnecessary. But that "enough v*airagya*" is not there. It is better to move on a disciplined path, step by step, so you don't become a victim of any accident. Accidents have happened, the possibility is there.

Many systems are working in the world, but there is no system as perfect as Patanjali's because no country has worked for so long. And Patanjali is not the originator of this system, he is only the systematizer. The system was developed for thousands of years before Patanjali; many people worked. Patanjali has given just the essence of thousands of years' work. But he has made it in such a way that you can move safely.

Just because you are moving inward, don't think that you are moving in a safe world. It can be unsafe. It is dangerous also, you can be lost in it. And if you are lost in it you will be mad. That's why teachers like Krishnamurti, who insist that no teacher is needed, are dangerous, because people who are uninitiated may take their standpoint and may start working on their own.

Remember, even if your wristwatch goes wrong, you have the tendency and the curiosity – because it comes from the monkeys – to open it and do something. It is difficult to resist it. You cannot believe that you don't know anything about it. You may be the owner, but just by being the owner of the watch doesn't mean you know anything. Don't open it! It is better to take it to the person who knows. And a watch is a simple mechanism. The mind is such a complex mechanism: never open it on your own because whatsoever you do will be wrong.

Sometimes it happens that your watch has gone wrong, you just shake it and it starts, but that is not a science. Sometimes it happens that something you do, and just by luck, accident, you feel something happening. But you have not become a master. And if it has happened once, don't try it again, because if you next shake your watch it may stop. This is not a science.

Don't move by accidents. Discipline is only a safeguard. Don't move by accidents! Move with a master who knows what he is doing. And he knows if something goes wrong he can bring it to the right path: one who is aware of your past and who is also aware of your future, and who can join together your past and future.

That is why there is so much emphasis on masters in Indian teachings. And they knew, and they meant it, because there is no mechanism as complex as the human mind, no computer as complex as the human mind.

Man has not yet been able to evolve anything comparable to the mind, and I think it is not ever going to be evolved, because who will evolve it? If the human mind can evolve something, it is always going to be lower and lesser than the mind that creates it. At least one thing is certain: that whatsoever the human mind creates, that created thing cannot create a human mind. So the human mind remains the superior-most, the supreme-most complex mechanism.

Don't do anything just because of curiosity or just because others are doing it. Get initiated, and move with someone who knows the path well. Otherwise madness can be the result. And it has happened before; it is happening to many people right now.

Patanjali doesn't believe in accidents, he believes in a scientific order. So he has given one-by-one steps. These two he makes his base: *vairagya*, desirelessness, and *abhyasa*, constant, conscious inner practice. *Abhyasa* is the means and *vairagya* is the goal. Desirelessness is the goal and constant, conscious inner practice is the means.

But the goal starts from the very beginning and the ends are hidden in the beginning. The tree is hidden in the seed, so the beginning implies the end. That's why he says desirelessness is needed in the beginning also. The beginning has the end in it and the end will also have the beginning in it.

So even when a master has become complete, total, he continues practicing. This will look absurd to you. You have to practice because you are in the beginning and the goal has not been achieved – but when the goal is achieved, even then the practice continues. It now becomes spontaneous, but it continues. It never stops. It cannot, because the end and the beginning are not two things. If the tree is in the seed, then in the tree again seeds will come.

One of Buddha's disciples, Purnakashyap asked, "We see, *bhante,* that you still follow a certain discipline."

Buddha? ...still following a certain discipline? He moves in a certain way, he sits in a certain way, he remains alert, he eats certain things, he behaves – everything seems to be disciplined.

So Purnakashyap said, "You have become enlightened, but we feel that you still have a certain discipline."

Buddha said, "It has become so ingrained that now I am not following it, it is following me. It has become a shadow. I need not think about it. It is there, always there. It has become a shadow."

So the end is in the beginning and the beginning will also be in the end. These are not two things, but two poles of one phenomenon.

Enough for today.

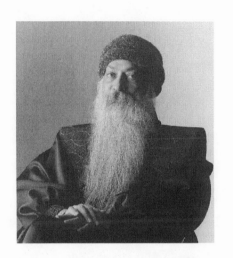

About Osho

Osho defies categorization. His thousands of talks cover everything from the individual quest for meaning to the most urgent social and political issues facing society today. Osho's books are not written but are transcribed from audio and video recordings of his extemporaneous talks to international audiences. As he puts it, "So remember: whatever I am saying is not just for you... I am talking also for the future generations."

Osho has been described by *The Sunday Times* in London as one of the "1000 Makers of the 20th Century" and by American author Tom Robbins as "the most dangerous man since Jesus Christ." *Sunday Mid-Day* (India) has selected Osho as one of ten people – along with Gandhi, Nehru and Buddha – who have changed the destiny of India.

About his own work Osho has said that he is helping to create the conditions for the birth of a new kind of human being. He often characterizes this new human being as "Zorba the Buddha" – capable both of enjoying the earthy pleasures of a Zorba the Greek and the silent serenity of a Gautama the Buddha.

Running like a thread through all aspects of Osho's talks and meditations is a vision that encompasses both the timeless wisdom of all ages past and the highest potential of today's (and tomorrow's) science and technology.

Osho is known for his revolutionary contribution to the science of inner transformation, with an approach to meditation that acknowledges the accelerated pace of contemporary life. His unique OSHO Active Meditations are designed to first release the accumulated stresses of body and mind, so that it is then easier to take an experience of stillness and thought-free relaxation into daily life.

Two autobiographical works by the author are available:
Autobiography of a Spiritually Incorrect Mystic,
St Martins Press, New York (book and eBook)
Glimpses of a Golden Childhood,
OSHO Media International, Pune, India

OSHO International Meditation Resort

Location
Located 100 miles southeast of Mumbai in the thriving modern city of Pune, India, the OSHO International Meditation Resort is a holiday destination with a difference. The Meditation Resort is spread over 28 acres of spectacular gardens in a beautiful tree-lined residential area.

Uniqueness
Each year the Meditation Resort welcomes thousands of people from more than 100 countries. The unique campus provides an opportunity for a direct personal experience of a new way of living – with more awareness, relaxation, celebration and creativity. A great variety of around-the-clock and around-the-year program options are available. Doing nothing and just relaxing is one of them!

All programs are based on the OSHO vision of "Zorba the Buddha" – a qualitatively new kind of human being who is able *both* to participate creatively in everyday life *and* to relax into silence and meditation.

OSHO Meditations
A full daily schedule of meditations for every type of person includes methods that are active and passive, traditional and revolutionary, and in particular the OSHO Active Meditations™. The meditations take place in what must be the world's largest meditation hall, the OSHO Auditorium.

OSHO Multiversity
Individual sessions, courses and workshops cover everything from creative arts to holistic health, personal transformation, relationship and life transition, work-as-meditation, esoteric sciences, and the "Zen" approach to sports and recreation. The secret of the OSHO Multiversity's success lies in the fact that all its programs are combined with meditation, supporting the understanding that as human beings we are far more than the sum of our parts.

OSHO Basho Spa

The luxurious Basho Spa provides for leisurely open-air swimming surrounded by trees and tropical green. The uniquely styled, spacious Jacuzzi, the saunas, gym, tennis courts...all these are enhanced by their stunningly beautiful setting.

Cuisine

A variety of different eating areas serve delicious Western, Asian and Indian vegetarian food – most of it organically grown especially for the Meditation Resort. Breads and cakes are baked in the resort's own bakery.

Night life

There are many evening events to choose from – dancing being at the top of the list! Other activities include full-moon meditations beneath the stars, variety shows, music performances and meditations for daily life.

Or you can just enjoy meeting people at the Plaza Café, or walking in the nighttime serenity of the gardens of this fairytale environment.

Facilities

You can buy all your basic necessities and toiletries in the Galleria. The Multimedia Gallery sells a large range of OSHO media products. There is also a bank, a travel agency and a Cyber Café on-campus. For those who enjoy shopping, Pune provides all the options, ranging from traditional and ethnic Indian products to all of the global brand-name stores.

Accommodation

You can choose to stay in the elegant rooms of the OSHO Guesthouse, or for longer stays opt for one of the OSHO Living-In program packages. Additionally there is a plentiful variety of nearby hotels and serviced apartments.

www.osho.com/meditationresort
www.osho.com/guesthouse
www.osho.com/livingin

For More Information

www. OSHO .com

a comprehensive multi-language website including a magazine, OSHO Books, OSHO Talks in audio and video formats, the OSHO Library text archive in English and Hindi and extensive information about OSHO Meditations. You will also find the program schedule of the OSHO Multiversity and information about the OSHO International Meditation Resort.

http://OSHO.com/AllAboutOSHO
http://OSHO.com/Resort
http://OSHO.com/Shop
http://www.youtube.com/OSHO
http://www.Twitter.com/OSHO
http://www.facebook.com/pages/OSHO.International

To contact OSHO International Foundation:
www.osho.com/oshointernational,
oshointernational@oshointernational.com

29050790R00141

Made in the USA
Lexington, KY
14 January 2014